Quantitative Methods for the Evaluation of Cancer Screening

Quantitative Methods for the Evaluation of Cancer Screening

Edited by

Stephen W. Duffy
Imperial Cancer Research Fund, London, UK

Catherine Hill
Institut Gustave Roussy, Villejuif, France

Jacques Estève
Centre Hospitalier Lyon-Sud, Pierre Benite, France

A member of the Hodder Headline Group
London
Co-published in the United States of America by
Oxford University Press Inc., New York

First published in Great Britain in 2001 by
Arnold, a member of the Hodder Headline Group,
338 Euston Road, London NW1 3BH

http://www.arnoldpublishers.com

Co-published in the United States of America by
Oxford University Press Inc.,
198 Madison Avenue, New York, NY10016

British Library Cataloguing in Publication Data
A catalogue record for this book is available from the British Library

Library of Congress Cataloging-in-Publication Data
A catalog record for this book is available from the Library of Congress

ISBN 0 340 74125 2 (hb)

1 2 3 4 5 6 7 8 9 10

Production Editor: Rada Radojicic
Production Controller: Bryan Eccleshall
Cover Design: Terry Griffiths

Typeset in 10pt Times by Replika Press Pvt Ltd, Delhi 110040, India
Printed and bound in Great Britain by MPG Books, Bodmin, Cornwall

What do you think about this book? Or any other Arnold title?
Please send your comments to feedback.arnold@hodder.co.uk

To our families

Contents

viii **Contents**

Contributors

Ariane Auquier
Department of Biostatistics and Epidemiology
Institut Gustave Roussy
Villejuif
FRANCE

Stuart G. Baker
Biometry Branch
National Cancer Institute
EPN 344
Bethesda MD
USA

Marjolein van Ballegooijen
Department of Public Health
Erasmus University
Rotterdam
NETHERLANDS

Rob Boer
Department of Public Health
Erasmus University
Rotterdam
NETHERLANDS

Hsiu-Hsi Chen
Graduate Institute of Epidemiology
College of Public Health
National Taiwan University
Taipei
TAIWAN

Jack Cuzick
Department of Mathematics, Statistics and
Epidemiology
Imperial Cancer Research Fund
Lincoln's Inn Fields
London
UK

Nicholas E. Day
Strangeways Research Laboratory
Cambridge
UK

Stephen W. Duffy
Department of Mathematics, Statistics and
Epidemiology
Imperial Cancer Research Fund
Lincoln's Inn Fields
London
UK

Jacques Estève
Biostatistics
Batiment 1M
Centre Hospitalier Lyon-Sud
Pierre Benite
FRANCE

Daniela Giorgi
Unit of Clinical and Descriptive
Epidemiology
Centre for the Study and Prevention of Cancer
Florence
ITALY

Timo Hakulinen
Finnish Cancer Registry
Institute for Statistical and Epidemiological
Cancer Research
Helsinki
FINLAND

Catherine Hill
Department of Biostatistics and Epidemiology
Institut Gustave Roussy
Villejuif
FRANCE

Harry J. de Koning
Department of Public Health
Erasmus University
Rotterdam
NETHERLANDS

Serge Koscielny
Department of Biostatistics and Epidemiology
Institut Gustave Roussy
Villejuif
FRANCE

Guy Launoy
Registre des Cancers Digestifs du Calvados
(CJF INSERM No. 9603)
Faculté de médecine
Caen
FRANCE

Jenny McCann
Cancer Intelligence Unit
Strangeways Research Laboratory
Cambridge
UK

Paul J. van der Maas
Department of Public Health
Erasmus University
Rotterdam
NETHERLANDS

Eugenio Paci
Unit of Clinical and Descriptive
Epidemiology
Centre for the Study and
Prevention of Cancer
Florence
ITALY

Teresa C. Prevost
MRC Biostatistics Unit
Institute of Public Health
University Forvie Site
Cambridge
UK

Marco Rosselli del Turco
Unit of Clinical and Descriptive
Epidemiology
Centre for the Study and
Prevention of Cancer
Florence
ITALY

Peter D. Sasieni
Department of Mathematics, Statistics and
Epidemiology
Imperial Cancer Research Fund
Lincoln's Inn Fields
London
UK

Diane Stockton
Scottish Cancer Surveillance Group
Information and Statistics Division
Scottish NHS
Edinburgh
UK

Laszlo Tabar
Mammography Department
Central Hospital
Falun
SWEDEN

Stephen D. Walter
McMaster University
Department of Clinical Epidemiology and
Biostatistics
Health Sciences Centre 2C16
Hamilton
CANADA

Ming-Fang Yen
Graduate Institute of Epidemiology
College of Public Health
National Taiwan University
Taipei
TAIWAN

Preface

This book grew out of a workshop in Paris in 1997, organised by the Institut National de la Santé et de la Recherche Médicale (INSERM), to which organisation considerable thanks are due. In particular, the editors would like to thank INSERM staff members Anne-Marie Laffaye and Claude Secco. Thanks are also due to various institutes whose facilities were used in the editing process. In particular, we thank the Institut Gustave Roussy, Paris, the Medical Research Council Biostatistics Unit, Cambridge, and the Research and Development Department of Papworth Hospital, Papworth Everard, UK. Authors of the various chapters acknowledge the advice, support or co-operation of the following individuals: E.A. Clarke, Lin Clegg, M. Gignoux, Matti Hakama, J. Hatcher, A. Newman, Richard Nixon, Lorna Saint-Ange, Linda Sharples, L.W. Stitt, A. Valla, and Neil Walker. Chapter authors also wish to thank the following bodies: the National Health Service Executive Eastern Region, the East Anglian Cancer Registry, the seven breast screening units and three health authorities of East Anglia, the staff and participants of the Swedish Two-County Trial of Mammographic Screening for Breast Cancer, the Association pour le Dépistage du Neuroblastome (ADN) and the Study Group for the Evaluation of Neuroblastoma Screening in Europe (SENSE).

Editing this book was an educative process for the three of us. The chapters gave us new insights on a range of approaches to design and analysis in evaluation of cancer screening programmes, and brought to our attention numerous issues in screening for cancers of the breast, cervix and large bowel. The authors were given a relatively free hand in drafting their chapters. The only constraint was a request that although there should be sufficient technical detail for the reader to try the approaches described, the emphasis should be on application, in order that the material be accessible to a range of professionals working in disease control and public health, as well as to statisticians and epidemiologists. The editors thank the authors for complying with this request. It is our hope that the material here proves as enlightening to the reader as it did to us.

Stephen W. Duffy
Catherine Hill
Jacques Estève

1

Introduction and brief history of cancer screening evaluation techniques

Stephen W. Duffy, Jacques Estève, Catherine Hill and Nicholas E. Day

1.1 Fundamental principles of cancer screening

Screening for disease can take place for a variety of reasons: to be effective, quarantine of cases of an infectious disease should include all contagious cases, including occult cases which need to be identified by screening; or in an immunisation programme, it might be necessary to first screen out those already infected. Another role for screening is to detect disease at a phase in its development in which successful treatment is more likely. This last aim is usually the target of a cancer screening programme. For many cancers, there is a strong dependence of survival on the stage of disease as measured by size of the primary tumour or indications of regional spread of the disease. For such cancers, there is at least a possibility that early detection of the cancer might prevent some late-stage tumours and hence reduce future rates of death from the disease. A striking example of this is cancer of the female breast. Figure 1.1 shows survival from breast cancer in a series of 2294 women with invasive breast cancer, by size of the tumour (Tabar *et al.*, 1992). Clearly the difference in survival by tumour size is considerable, greater than could be achieved by variations in therapy. Observations of this kind gave rise to the idea of detecting the disease early, and hence while the tumour is smaller and less potentially fatal.

For cancers at other sites, there are recognised premalignant conditions whose presence indicates a strong possibility of the cancer developing in the near future, and which are amenable to treatment to prevent the occurrence of cancer at the site at all. An example of this is cervical cancer, which may be preceded by cervical intraepithelial neoplasia. This can be treated surgically before the occurrence of invasive cervical carcinoma, forestalling the development of the disease. Similar examples might be adenomatous

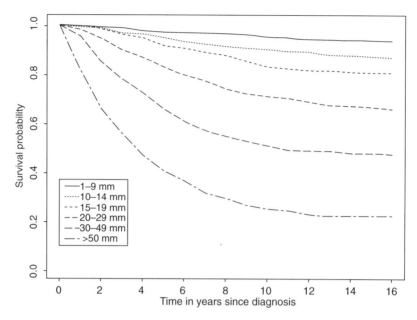

Figure 1.1 Survival of 2294 invasive breast cancer patients by size of tumour

polyp of the large bowel as a precursor of large bowel cancer, or oral leukoplakia as a premalignant oral condition.

Some cancers are known to be strongly associated with certain infectious agents. The human papilloma virus is arguably the major causal factor for cervical carcinoma. Very high rates of nasopharyngeal cancer are known to occur in subjects positive for an Epstein–Barr virus reactivation phase. Liver cancer is strongly associated with Hepatitis B virus. For such cancers, if a strong effect of disease stage was observed on survival, a possible strategy might be a two-stage screening programme. The first stage would be population screening by serological tests for the infectious agent, and the second direct screening for preclinical cancer only in those with positive serological results.

The above illustrates that there is in theory a wide range of malignancies which are potentially amenable to screening. In practice, however, rigorous examination of the disease, the potential screening tool, and the public health context, are necessary before even considering experimentation with screening. Often cited are the Wilson and Jungner (1968) criteria, a list of ten principles which a disease and a potential screening tool should satisfy. With hindsight, these criteria can be seen as incomplete (they do not explicitly include the condition that disease detected at an early stage should be more successfully treatable than disease detected later), and indeed contentious (they include the condition that the natural history of the disease should be adequately understood, something which is still not true of cancers of the breast or cervix, which are demonstrably amenable to screening). They do, however, help us to focus on the major issues surrounding the decision of whether screening is at least worth investigating in principle. Essentially the disease should be an important health problem, there should be a preclinical state which is more amenable to successful treatment than clinical disease, and there should be an acceptable screening instrument for detection of the disease in this preclinical state.

Acceptability of the screening instrument encompasses effectiveness of detection (see Section 1.2 below), safety and comfort of the persons screened, and cost. There is general agreement that these are necessary, although not sufficient conditions for screening to be useful.

The ultimate goal of a cancer screening programme is to prevent deaths from the disease (although this is sometimes achieved as in the case of cervical cancer by preventing the disease from occurring at all). The ideal method of evaluation would therefore be the comparison of deaths from the cancer in question in an unscreened population with deaths in a population screened for that cancer. This is usually a viable option only in the context of a randomised controlled trial. Outside of the randomised trial environment, alternative quantitative tools are required to at least give some estimate of the likely effect on mortality. In addition, there is a need for methods which may be used in a diagnostic context on a population screening programme, not only to detect whether the programme is on target to reduce deaths from the disease but also to point to the reasons for any deficiency (poor sensitivity, inappropriate interval between screens, poor compliance, and so on). It is the purpose of this book to draw together expert knowledge on the methods available, and to demonstrate the use of these methods in practice. In the remainder of this chapter, we shall define the basic measures which the methods aim to estimate.

1.2 Direct indicators of effectiveness of screening for cancer

Returning to the randomised trial environment to demonstrate the ideal indicator of effectiveness, we define the mortality rate ratio as

$$RR = \frac{D_s/P_s}{D_c/P_c}$$

where D_s and P_s are the numbers of deaths from the cancer screened for and person-years at risk, respectively, in the group randomised to invitation to screening and D_c and P_c are the corresponding figures in the control group randomised to no such invitation. If screening were effective in reducing mortality, the rate ratio would be smaller than 1.0. Note that this is based on mortality, the number of deaths from the disease in the population as a whole, not case survival from diagnosis of the disease. In a screening study, the latter is biased by the fact that if a case is detected by screening, say a year earlier than it would have been if left to develop to the clinical phase, then the survival is tautologically increased by one year even if the early detection confers no benefit (lead time bias), and potentially by increased diagnosis of relatively indolent cases by screening (length bias).

Let us now define as informally as possible a few statistical terms. A significant effect observed from empirical data is one which is unlikely, by a given criterion, to be compatible with chance. The usual criterion used is the 5% significance level, that is, we conclude that our results are not compatible with chance if the probability of our observed results, or results more extreme than these, is less than 0.05 under the assumption of pure chance and no real effect. Thus for example it would be relevant to test whether an observed rate ratio was significantly different from unity (i.e. whether there was a difference between the death rate of the invited group and that of the control group which was not compatible with pure chance).

A 95% confidence interval is an estimated range within which we estimate the true value of a parameter to lie, giving a range of plausible values compatible with the uncertainty in our data. A basic rule is that the smaller the amount of data available, the greater the uncertainty and the wider the confidence interval.

Statistical methods are readily available to test whether a mortality rate ratio differs significantly from unity, to calculate a 95% confidence interval on the rate ratio and to take into account the effect of possible covariables, such as age (Breslow and Day, 1987). For example, it is not uncommon to see the results of a randomised trial of screening as Tabar *et al.* (1992) reported on the Swedish Two-County Trial of breast cancer screening as a breast cancer mortality rate ratio of 0.70, with a 95% confidence interval of (0.58–0.85), together with a table of deaths from breast cancer and person-years at risk in both the invited and control groups.

In reality, the job of evaluating disease screening is more complex than this. Even if we have mortality data from a randomised trial, there are other factors to consider, such as the sensitivity and specificity of the screening tool, financial and human costs, and uptake of the screening by the population. It is reasonable, however, to take this randomised comparison of mortality rates as the ideal, in the sense that if no lives are saved by the screening, it is not worth doing and therefore other measures are unnecessary, except perhaps as a means to establish why the screening is not working.

Once randomised trials have been carried out, if they do indicate a benefit from screening in terms of mortality, one might be forgiven for thinking that service screening can then be applied without further evaluation. However, success is only guaranteed if the screening quality in the randomised trials is reproduced in the subsequent service screening programmes, and to justify the resources expended it is necessary to monitor the screening to ensure that this quality is achieved and maintained. This is analogous to post-marketing surveillance of drugs which have already undergone successful clinical trial. It is arguable that there are more features capable of failure in delivery of a screening service than in the prescription of a new antibiotic, and therefore the evaluation of the former is likely to be more complex.

The fundamental aim of evaluation of a cancer screening programme outwith a randomised trial is therefore to estimate the likely benefit in terms of a mortality reduction without a randomised comparator group, with the secondary purpose of assessing whether improvements to the design or quality of the screening service are necessary. A mortality effect can be estimated by comparing mortality before and after the initiation of screening. This may be biased by increased disease ascertainment with screening, in that the knowledge that a person dying of another cause has a history of cancer may make it more likely that that cancer will appear as a contributory factor on the death certificate. It may also be confounded with changes in therapeutic practice over time. If screening is introduced in different regions at different times, it may be that a contemporaneous mortality comparison is possible, which is still prone to ascertainment bias, but not to confounding with other temporal changes. To avoid ascertainment bias, we might compare excess mortality, that is the numbers of deaths among breast cancer cases after elimination of the expected numbers of deaths in these cases from causes other than breast cancer (Lenner and Jonsson, 1997). A major problem with any strategy involving actual mortality is that reliable mortality statistics are unlikely to be available until several years after the inception of the screening programme, and providers of screening need to know if it is likely to be effective before the mortality results are available, in order to take early action to rectify deficiencies in the programme.

1.3 Indirect indicators of effectiveness and diagnostic benchmarks

Evaluation therefore requires early indicators of whether a screening programme is predicted to deliver the desired mortality reduction and of the reasons for a likely failure to do so. To illustrate the issues involved, let us consider breast and cervical screening in turn. To take first the example of mammographic screening for breast cancer, there are some solutions readily available, partly from knowledge of the disease natural history and secondly from the considerable volume of information published from randomised trials of breast cancer screening. It has already been noted that there is a strong gradient of survival with size of the primary tumour in breast cancer. Indeed, as with many other tumours there is a strong effect of measures of stage on prognosis. Successful reduction in mortality by screening for breast cancer is invariably preceded by a reduction in the incidence of tumours of advanced stage (see Table 1.1). It has also been established that predicted mortality from the size, node status (whether the cancer has invaded the regional lymph nodes) and malignancy grade (a histological measure of aggressive potential of the tumour) correlates well with observed mortality in the randomised trials of breast cancer screening. Therefore, a primary element of evaluation of a breast cancer screening programme has to be the effect of the programme on incidence of the disease by stage. This has the advantages over actual mortality that it is available earlier and that before screening–after screening comparisons are not confounded by changes in therapy over time.

It is also usually necessary to quantify the manner in which the screening is working (or not working), in order to maintain quality and improve matters if the screening is deficient in any area. Further evaluation should aim at establishing penetration of screening to the target population, sensitivity and specificity of the screening and their implications for delayed diagnosis, unnecessary investigations and procedures in healthy subjects (involving both human and health services resource costs) and stage at diagnosis. It is important that such evaluation is performed in the light of knowledge of the natural history of the disease and of the screening process designed to interrupt this natural history.

Figure 1.2 shows the assumed course of disease in relation to screening. Before time t_0, there is no detectable disease. From t_0 onwards the disease is detectable by screening. At t_1 the disease becomes symptomatic and is diagnosed clinically. The difference $t_1 - t_0$, is the duration of the preclinical screen-detectable period, known as the sojourn time. If a screen occurs, detecting the cancer at t_2, then $t_1 - t_2$ is known as the lead time. During the preclinical detectable period a breast tumour is growing with respect to size, potential

Table 1.1 Relative mortality from breast cancer and relative incidence of tumours at stage II or worse, by age group, in the Swedish Two-County Trial of breast cancer screening

Age group	Relative mortality (invited vs control)	Relative incidence Stage II+ (invited vs control)
40–49	0.87	0.84
50–59	0.66	0.62
60–69	0.60	0.61
70–74	0.79	0.88

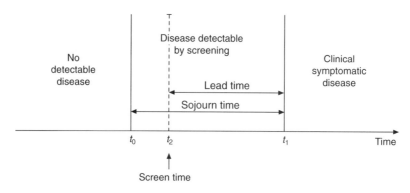

Figure 1.2 A simple representation of the course of disease as related to screening

invasion of the lymph nodes and, according to recent research findings, the malignancy grade. Thus the earlier the tumour is diagnosed during the preclinical period, the better will be the prognosis for the patient. The potential of the screening programme to detect the tumour early will depend on the sojourn time, the frequency of screening and the sensitivity of the screening tool. Note that we are aiming here not to prevent breast cancers from occurring, but simply to detect them at an earlier phase in the natural history.

Now, consider the process of screening for breast cancer. The usual procedure is as follows. Asymptomatic women from the general population are invited to mammography, an X-ray of the breast. A certain proportion of them will accept the invitation. For those who do so, the vast majority will have no suspicious features on the mammogram, but a small proportion will have features which may be related to malignancy. This latter group will be recalled for further assessment, which may take the form of physical examination of the breasts, further mammography, including micromagnification, ultrasound examination, and fine needle aspiration. Of these, a proportion will be diagnosed with malignancy or as very likely to have malignancy and will be referred for surgery to remove the malignancy. After surgery, the excised tissue will undergo histopathological examination and a definitive diagnosis will be available.

Clearly then, we require firstly to assess the effect of the programme on incidence of the tumours by size, node status and malignancy grade, to estimate participation rates in the population, rates of recall, surgery and cancer in those who do attend, and sensitivity and specificity of the screening. Sensitivity is defined as the probability that if a tumour in the preclinical screen-detectable phase is subjected to screening then it is diagnosed as a result of that screening. Specificity is the probability that a person free of disease is not diagnosed as having the disease as a result of the screening. In a sense this should always be 100%, since almost 100% of tumours will be confirmed by histology. There is, however, a possibility that screening may diagnose tumours which would never have surfaced clinically had no screening taken place. It should be noted that specificity of the initial test is usually very low in a screening programme. Recall for assessment after a suspicious mammogram is not a positive diagnosis of any disease, simply an indication that further diagnostic work is needed.

Since only the subjects who are identified by the programme actually undergo definitive histological diagnosis, estimation of sensitivity and specificity are not as straightforward as in a designed experiment on a new diagnostic tool, where all subjects undergo definitive diagnosis. To determine disease in those who are screened negative, we therefore need to follow up the subjects screened negative for cancers which occur clinically between screens (interval cancers).

If sensitivity is good, one would expect the rate of interval cancers in the year immediately after a screen to be small in comparison with the incidence rate in the absence of screening, since the screen will already have diagnosed the cancers which would have arisen clinically. In order to estimate the proportion of cancers missed at a screen, it is necessary to know how many of the interval cancers have genuinely entered and subsequently left the preclinical period since the screen, and how many were already in the preclinical period at the time of the screen but were missed. Quantifying these two populations involves the underlying incidence of the disease and the average duration of the preclinical screen-detectable period (known usually as the mean sojourn time).

Table 1.2 shows a broad strategy of evaluation of a breast cancer screening programme. Models and methods for estimation of the quantities specified are available and will be the subject of several of the subsequent chapters.

Now, let us consider the case of cervical cancer screening. In a sense, the term cervical cancer screening is a misnomer, since the objective is to find a premalignant condition, or at worst cervical carcinoma *in situ*, treat this condition and thus prevent invasive cervical cancer from occurring. The basic physical procedure is that a smear is taken from the cervix, and cytological examination of the smear material is taken to identify cellular changes which are likely to be associated with a malignant process. There are numerous ways of classifying cervical smears, but a simple and relevant classification is no suspicious features, mild dyskaryosis, moderate dyskaryosis, severe dyskaryosis and malignancy. Severe dyskaryosis is frequently associated with cervical carcinoma *in situ*, and would invariably lead to further investigation and various possible interventions. There is no universally agreed policy for mild and moderate dyskaryosis, although it is becoming more standard to order further investigation on observation of moderate dyskaryosis.

In this case, we are screening for a premalignant or preinvasive condition. In the absence of screening, some cases of the premalignant condition would have progressed to invasive cervical carcinoma and others would not. The progressive cases cannot be distinguished absolutely from the non-progressive. Table 1.3 shows the proportions of smears with severe dyskaryosis or worse by English region in 1993–94, with the corresponding incidence rates of invasive cervical cancer in 1974, as a measure of the underlying incidence of disease. Note first that the abnormal smears are only modestly correlated with the incidence rates. Note also that the prevalence of severe dyskaryotic or worse smears is some 50 times the underlying incidence of invasive cervical carcinoma. The premalignant condition associated with severe dyskaryosis is known to have a long duration before invasive carcinoma occurs, but even assuming a duration of 10 years, and therefore a prevalence at screening of around 10 times the invasive carcinoma incidence, one would still expect the majority of severe dyskaryosis cases not to progress to malignancy.

Thus the mechanism of a screening's effect in the case of cervical cancer is fundamentally different from that of screening for breast cancer, and evaluation measures must also be different. Because of the long premalignant period and the relative rarity of invasive cervical carcinoma in most developed countries (made rarer still if the screening is successful), any informative evaluation based on observed mortality from the disease will not be apparent until a decade or so after the screening commences. Clearly the incidence

Table 1.2 Components of evaluation of a breast cancer screening programme

Type of measure	Measure	Target of measure
Basic observation	Rates of attendance by age and time	Acceptability to the population, likely population effect
	Rates of recall for assessment, cytology, surgery and cancer detection by age and time	Screening and diagnostic quality
	Cancer detection rates by age, size, node status and malignancy grade	Sensitivity by phase of development of tumour
	Interval cancer incidence by age and time since last screen	Effectiveness of early detection
	Rates of cancer in attenders and non-attenders, by age, size, lymph node status and malignancy grade	Likely benefit taking account of selection bias
Modelled estimates	Sojourn time, lead time, test sensitivity and programme sensitivity, by age and time	Effectiveness of early detection, identification of causes of any deficiencies
	Comparison of expected prevalence based on sojourn time and sensitivity with observed prevalence at first and subsequent screens	Over-diagnosis
	Incidence in screened population compared with expected incidence in the absence of screening, by histology and other tumour attributes	Over-diagnosis of specific types of tumour (e.g. ductal carcinoma *in situ*)
	Projected deaths from breast cancer based on size, node status and malignancy grade of tumours diagnosed, compared with that expected in the absence of screening	Prediction of mortality benefit
Direct indicators of effect of screening	Projection of anticipated mortality from breast cancer if screening had not been introduced compared to observed mortality since screening began	Estimation of mortality benefit – confounded by changes in therapy and ascertainment bias
	Projection of anticipated incidence of advanced tumours if screening had not been introduced compared to observed incidence since screening began	Prediction of mortality benefit – confounded by ascertainment bias
	Excess mortality from breast cancer before and after the start of screening	Estimation of mortality benefit – confounded by changes in therapy

of invasive cervical carcinoma is a reliable indicator of the success of the programme – if the incidence is reduced following the initiation of a screening programme, this is evidence that the programme is indeed detecting lesions at a preinvasive stage and preventing the occurrence of invasive cancer. This has been used to demonstrate a beneficial effect of a dramatic increase in the coverage rate of cervical screening in East Anglia, UK, in the late 1980s (Gibson *et al.*, 1997).

Table 1.3 Cervical smears with severe dyskaryosis or worse in 1993–94, and incidence of invasive cervical cancer in 1974, by English region

Region	Severe dyskaryosis or worse per 1000 women screened 1993–94[a]	Incidence per 1000 of invasive cervical carcinoma, 1974[b]
SE Thames	5	0.15
Wessex	6	0.20
Yorkshire	6	0.17
Trent	6	0.18
East Anglia	6	0.16
West Midlands	6	0.14
Oxford	6	0.14
NW Thames	7	0.13
NE Thames	8	0.10
SW Thames	8	0.12
Northern	9	0.16
South West	10	0.16
Mersey	11	0.18
North West	12	0.21

[a]Source: Department of Health, 1995.
[b]Source: Office of Population Censuses and Surveys, 1980.

Other possible indicators of the quality of a cervical screening programme include coverage rates, proportion of inadequate smears, proportion of abnormal smears in relation to final diagnosis, colposcopy and other assessment rates in relation to final diagnosis, biopsy results compared to smear test results, and inter- and intra-laboratory quality control estimates from repeat cytology on the same smears. Because the natural history of the premalignant condition screened for is not well understood, however, there are no universal standards with which to compare most of these measures, and interpretation has to be fairly tentative.

The above illustrates the complexity of the task of evaluation. The subsequent chapters will illustrate some of the methods of dealing with this complexity.

1.4 Historical and bibliographic notes on cancer screening evaluation

The first randomised controlled trial evidence on the effect of cancer screening on mortality from the disease in question was the Health Insurance Plan of Greater New York (HIP) Study of breast cancer screening (Shapiro *et al.*, 1971). Methodological research on modelling the mechanism of screening, however, predates this, the seminal work being by Zelen and Feinleib (1969). Zelen and Feinleib developed a model with an exponential distribution of time spent in the preclinical phase. This has been used as the fundamental building block in numerous subsequent modelling approaches (for a review, see Stevenson, 1995). Other early influential temporal modelling approaches include those of Prorok (1976), Eddy (1980) and Walter and Day (1983), all of which draw on Zelen and Feinleib's original work. More recently, as methods and software for modelling have become more advanced, the models themselves have become more ambitious, incorporating variables representing or influencing tumour progression and formal prediction of subsequent deaths from the disease. Two major approaches are computer simulation of disease incidence, progression, fatality and screening intervention (Van den Akker-Van Marle et al., 1997), and empirical estimation from screening programmes of tumour progression parameters and the arrest of such progression by early detection (Chen et al., 1997a, b). Elements of both approaches will appear in subsequent chapters.

For purposes of less mathematically formal evaluation, early techniques emphasised the incidence of disease after a screen (interval cancers), applied to evaluation of screening for cancer at any anatomical site (Shapiro et al., 1974; Walter and Day, 1983; Prorok and Miller, 1984; Hakama et al., 1986). Clearly, immediately after a population has been screened, the incidence of disease should fall as a result of cancers anticipated by the screen. The extent to which such incidence falls is informative about the lead time achieved and the sensitivity of the test. Another long-established principle of evaluation is that where the aim of screening is to detect cancer at an earlier phase in its development screening should reduce the rates of disease at advanced stage. This was known in theory (Shwartz, 1978) and eloquently demonstrated in practice by the results of the Swedish Two-County Trial of screening for breast cancer (Tabar et al., 1985). The analogous phenomenon where screening is for a precursor of cancer, as in the case of cervical carcinoma, is that screening should reduce the rate of cancer in the population screened. This has also been long established (Lundin et al., 1965; Hakama et al., 1986).

In terms of study design for evaluation, three major design strategies are commonly used. The first is the randomised controlled trial, which has been used to assess screening for cancers of the breast (for a review, see Organizing Committee and Collaborators, 1996), lung (Berlin et al., 1984) and large bowel (Kronborg et al., 1996).

While the randomised trial is the ideal means to assess whether the screening can be made to work in principle, there remains the problem of evaluating a program in routine public health practice. This is often carried out by the uncontrolled cohort design, involving detailed follow-up of a cohort which is screened or offered screening, usually including estimation of disease incidence, stage and mortality, sometimes comparing stage and mortality before and after introduction of screening, and usually addressing incidence after a negative screen in some detail. This design strategy has been used in assessing the effects of screening for cancers at many sites, but to greatest effect in evaluation of cervical cancer screening (Hakama et al., 1986).

Another design frequently used to assess the effect of screening is a retrospective case-control design. For evaluation of breast cancer screening, deaths from breast cancer constitute the cases, women still alive constitute the controls, and the screening history of the two groups is compared (Palli et al., 1989). In the case of cervical cancer, cases of invasive cervical carcinoma are the cases, and women free of the disease are the controls (Macgregor et al., 1985). The design may be prone to bias, depending on what the study aims to estimate, and results must always be interpreted cautiously (Moss, 1991).

The extent to which a general evaluation procedure can be prescribed varies considerably among different cancer sites. For breast cancer, where there is a considerable body of data from randomised trials of screening and a reasonable understanding of the natural history and the screening process, general rules can be developed (Day et al., 1989). For tumours at other sites, the techniques and strategies are at a more developmental stage. It is the aim of the subsequent chapters of this book to enumerate the techniques available in the screening evaluator's toolbox and to demonstrate the use of some of the more important of these, in such a way that readers can then use the techniques on their own screening programmes.

References

Berlin, N.I., Buncher, C.R., Fontana, R.S., Frost, J.K. and Melamed, M.R. (1984). The National Cancer Institute Cooperative Early Lung Cancer Detection Program. *Amer. Rev. Respir. Dis.*, **130**, 545–9.

Breslow, N.E. and Day, N.E. (1987). *Statistical Methods in Cancer Research II: The Design and Analysis of Cohort Studies*. International Agency for Research on Cancer, Lyon.

Chen, H.H., Duffy, S.W., Tabar, L. and Day, N.E. (1997a). Markov chain models for progression of breast cancer. Part I: tumour attributes and the preclinical screen-detectable phase. *J. Epidemiol. Biostat*, **2**, 9–23.

Chen, H.H., Duffy, S.W., Tabar, L. and Day, N.E. (1997b). Markov chain models for progression of breast cancer. Part II: prediction of outcomes for different screening regimes. *J. Epidemiol. Biostat*, **2**, 25–35.

Day, N.E., Williams, D.R.R. and Khaw, K.T. (1989). Breast cancer screening programmes: the development of a monitoring and evaluation system. *Br. J. Cancer*, **59**, 954–8.

Department of Health, Statistics Division (1995). Form KC61 (Pathology Laboratory Activity). Department of Health, London.

Eddy, D. (1980). *Screening for Cancer: Theory, Analysis and Design*. Prentice-Hall, Englewood Cliffs.

Gibson, L., Spiegelhalter, D.J., Camilleri-Ferrante, C. and Day, N.E. (1997). Trends in cervical cancer incidence in East Anglia from 1971 to 1993. *J. Med. Screening*, **4**, 44–8.

Hakama, M., Miller, A.B. and Day, N.E. (1986). *Screening for Cancer of the Uterine Cervix*. International Agency for Research on Cancer, Lyon.

Kronborg, O., Fenger, C., Olsen, J., Jorgensen, O.D. and Sondergaard, O. (1996). Randomized study of screening for colorectal cancer with faecal-occult-blood test. *Lancet*, **348**, 1467–71.

Lenner, P. and Jonsson, H. (1997). Excess mortality from breast cancer in relation to mammography screening in northern Sweden. *J. Med. Screening*, **4**, 6–9.

Lundin, F.E., Christopherson, W.M., Mendez, W.M. and Parker, J.E. (1965). Morbidity from cervical cancer. Effects of cervical cytology and socioeconomic status. *J. Natl. Cancer Inst.*, **35**, 1015–25.

Macgregor, J.E., Moss, S.M., Parkin, D.M. and Day, N.E. (1985). A case-control study of cervical cancer screening in North-East Scotland. *Br. Med. J.*, **290**, 1543–6.

Moss, S.M. (1991). Case-control studies of screening. In: Miller, A.B., Chamberlain, J., Day, N.E., Hakama, M. and Prorok, P.C., eds, *Cancer Screening*. Cambridge University Press.

Office of Population Censuses and Surveys (1980). *Cancer Statistics: Registrations 1974*. Her Majesty's Stationery Office, London.

Organizing Committee and Collaborators, Falun Meeting (1996). Breast-cancer screening with mammography in women aged 40–49 years. *Int. J. Cancer*, **68**, 693–9.

Palli, D., Rosselli del Turco, M., Buiatti, E., Ciatto, S., Crocetti, E. and Paci, E. (1989). Time interval since last test in a breast cancer screening programme: a case-control study in Italy. *J. Epidemiol. Comm. Hlth.*, **43**, 241–8.

Prorok, P.C. (1976). The theory of periodic screening II: doubly bounded recurrence times and mean lead time and detection probability estimation. *Adv. App. Prob.*, **8**, 460–76.

Prorok, P.C. and Miller, A.B., eds (1984). *Screening for Cancer I: General Principles on Evaluation of Screening for Cancer and Screening for Lung, Bladder and Oral Cancer*. International Union Against Cancer, Geneva.

Shapiro, S., Strax, P. and Venet, L. (1971). Periodic breast cancer screening in reducing mortality from breast cancer. *J. Amer. Med. Assoc.*, **215**, 1777–85.

Shapiro, S., Goldberg, J.D. and Hutchison, G.B. (1974). Lead time in breast cancer detection and implications for periodicity of screening. *Amer. J. Epidemiol.*, **100**, 357–66.

Shwartz, M. (1978). A mathematical model used to analyze breast cancer screening strategies. *Operations Research*, **26**, 937–55.

Stevenson, C.E. (1995). Statistical models for cancer screening. *Statist. Meth. Med. Res.*, **4**, 18–32.

Tabar, L., Fagerberg, C.J.G., Gad, A., *et al.* (1985). Reduction in mortality from breast cancer after mass screening with mammography. *Lancet*, **i**, 829–32.

Tabar, L., Fagerberg, G., Duffy, S.W., Day, N.E., Gad, A. and Grontoft, O. (1992). Update of the Swedish two-county program of mammographic screening for breast cancer. *Radiol. Clin. N. Amer.*, **30**, 187–210.

Van den Akker-Van Marle, M.E., Reep-Van den Bergh, C.M.M., Boer, R., Del Moral, A., Ascunce, N. and de Koning, H.J. (1997). Breast cancer screening in Navarra: interpretation of a high detection rate at the first screening round and a low rate at the second round. *Int. J. Cancer*, **73**, 464–9.

Walter, S.D. and Day, N.E. (1983). Estimation of the duration of a preclinical disease state using screening data. *Amer. J. Epidemiol.*, **118**, 865–86.

Wilson, J.M.G. and Junger, G. (1968). *Principles and Practice of Screening for Disease*. World Health Organisation, Geneva.

Zelen, M. and Feinleib, M. (1969). On the theory of screening for chronic diseases. *Biometrika*, **56**, 601–13.

2

Important influences on effectiveness and costs to be considered in the evaluation of cancer screening

Rob Boer, Harry J. de Koning, Marjolein van Ballegooijen and Paul J. van der Maas

2.1 Introduction

Trials of cancer screening are designed to give an answer to the question of whether screening is effective, in particular in reducing cancer mortality. The main result of such a design is presented as a relative risk of dying from cancer in the study group (invited to screening) as compared to the control group (not invited). This relative risk is often treated as a constant which does not depend on the particular screening situation (Elwood *et al.*, 1993). But it has been shown that the cost-effectiveness ratio can differ strongly with economic context (Brown and Fintor, 1993). Besides the economic context, effectiveness and costs of screening also strongly depend on several other aspects of the screening situation. In this chapter we describe such aspects and give some examples of quantification of their influence as estimated with the aid of the MISCAN simulation package (Habbema *et al.*, 1985; Loeve *et al.*, 1999) with examples mainly from models of breast cancer screening (van Oortmarssen *et al.*, 1990; de Koning *et al.*, 1991; de Koning *et al.*, 1995), because international interest has focused strongly on screening for cancer of this site. Other examples are mostly from models of cervical cancer screening (van Ballegooijen *et al.*, 1990; Koopmanschap *et al.*, 1990; van Ballegooijen *et al.*, 1992a; van Ballegooijen *et al.*, 1995; van Ballegooijen *et al.*, 1997). Our models on prostate cancer screening (Boer *et al.*, 1997) and colorectal cancer screening (Loeve *et al.*, 1999) are not yet suitable for public health decision support because the evidence on efficacy is too preliminary for prostate cancer screening in general and for colorectal cancer screening if any screening modality other than faecal occult blood testing is to be considered.

Results from trials are essential for sensible public health decisions on cancer screening. In this chapter it is shown that they cannot automatically be extrapolated to population screening situations without taking into account epidemiology, demography, screening quality, policy and history, clinical practice and costs. The role of these components of a detailed evaluation of a screening programme are now described in more detail.

2.2 Epidemiology in the absence of screening

Two aspects of the epidemiology of different cancers are of major importance in this context. Firstly, it is important to determine the level of risk of a cancer by age which can be expressed by two measures: incidence and survival or mortality from that cancer. Secondly, the stage distribution in a situation without screening and the strongly related duration of the period in which tumours can be detected by screening are vital to the potential success of a screening programme. The potential number of cancer deaths prevented and life-years gained by screening is proportional, roughly speaking, to the level of risk of the cancer in question. Because the level of risk is very different among populations for which screening is considered, it is of great importance for the cost-effectiveness of screening. For instance in an analysis of the cost-effectiveness of breast cancer screening in different countries of the European Union, it was found that applying a similar screening strategy to both Spain and the United Kingdom resulted in an expected cost per life-year gained in the former more than twice as high as in the latter. This was mainly because the underlying mortality from breast cancer in the UK is approximately twice as high as in Spain (van Ineveld et al., 1993). Table 2.1 compares the crude rate of breast cancer mortality and number of life-years gained per 1000 screens and cost-effectiveness ratio estimated for similar screening programmes in Spain and in the UK.

For cervical cancer, differences in the level of risk depending on the region where screening is considered are even greater; the pattern of age distribution of the risk also varies strongly (Gustafsson et al., 1997). Besides substantial regional variation in risk, there can also be considerable variation over time. For instance, the risk of cervical cancer in the Netherlands appears to decrease considerably by birth cohort over past decades leading to a trend of decreasing mortality from cervical cancer over time prior to any substantial screening activity which might continue to occur without any screening effort. Therefore the effect of screening may be much smaller than would appear from the observed decrease in cervical cancer mortality (van Ballegooijen, 1998).

Stage distribution is also observed to differ strongly between populations. One can reasonably assume that cancer is usually a process in which one moves in one direction from relatively favourable stages to increasingly worse stages of the disease. A worse

Table 2.1 Relation between risk level and cost-effectiveness of a breast cancer screening programme (van Ineveld et al., 1993)

	Spain	UK
Mortality (crude rate per 100 000 women)	25	52
Life-years gained per 1000 screens	8.2	19.6
Cost per life-year gained (£/ly)	4900	2000

stage distribution therefore implies that on average the disease process has been going on for longer, and that the period of possible detection by screening may be longer.

A very good example of this for breast cancer screening can be found in and around the Italian city of Florence. After running the Florence District Programme in the areas around Florence (the District) for several years, the same executive group extended screening to within the City of Florence. While the breast cancer incidence in the City is about one and a half times higher than in the surrounding District, Table 2.2 shows that the detection rates at first screenings are only 15% higher (Paci *et al.*, 1995). This can be explained when one considers the poorer stage distribution in the District than in the City, before screening took place in either location. One might assume that the stage distribution in the absence of screening and the screen-detectable course of the disease are features of a Markov process in which the natural course of the disease is the same, although the time of diagnosis can be earlier or later. This would imply that transition rates for progression from one preclinical stage to the next are the same in the District and City, while the more favourable clinical stage distribution is observed in the City because of higher transition rates to clinical detection. This assumption would predict the screen-detectable preclinical period of the City to be 0.77 of that in the District, while the observed difference in prevalence/incidence ratio is 0.82, which seems close enough to support the assumption. A poorer stage distribution in association with longer potential lead times would arguably confer a larger probability of benefit for a woman taking part in screening, but might also be related to negative effects associated with lead time, especially a larger probability of detecting cancer which would not be detected in the absence of screening, due for example to death from other causes before symptomatic disease.

A poorer clinical stage distribution in the absence of screening should also lead to a higher detection rate at first screening, and to a somewhat larger difference between the stage distribution of screen-detected cases and that prevailing before screening started. Hence, a poorer clinical stage distribution is expected to lead to a larger extra demand for health care facilities for the primary therapy of cancer detected due to screening. For instance, there would almost certainly be an increase in the demand for radiotherapy at the start of a breast cancer screening programme and an even stronger increase in the number of diagnoses and treatments of non-palpable tumours requiring stereotactically guided biopsies.

Table 2.2 Association between prevalence/incidence ratio and stage distribution among clinically detected cases of breast cancer in and around Florence, Italy

	Florence District Programme	City of Florence
Incidence in age group 50–69 = I (per 1000)	1.6	2.3
Fraction T2+ cases diagnosed clinically before screening	61%	42%
Detection rate at prevalence screen (per 1000) = P	6.4	7.4
P/I	3.9	3.2

2.3 Demography

Demography describes the size of the population, the age and sex distribution of the population and total mortality. The major influence of demography is obvious: the size of the population is proportional to the total effects in numbers and costs of a screening programme and therefore relates to the logistics and financing of the programme, especially at its initiation. Population size is not of great influence on efficiency (the cost-effectiveness ratio) of the programme, as there are usually only minor scale effects. The age distribution of the population in which screening is performed can have an important influence: in general a younger population leads to finding fewer cancers, but to a larger number of life-years gained per cancer death prevented by the programme. Total mortality is also of influence, since a lower life expectancy at a given age leads to fewer possible life-years gained by preventing cancer death, and to a higher probability of detecting a cancer at screening which would not have been diagnosed or would not have led to dying from the cancer in question in the absence of screening.

However, when comparing different geographical areas in which a breast cancer screening programme is being implemented or considered, demography will probably not be of overriding influence on cost-effectiveness since no major differences are to be expected concerning age distribution and total mortality between areas of the developed world, while in the developing countries, mass screening for breast cancer is not (yet) a serious option. The situation is rather different when screening for cervical cancer is considered. For cervical cancer, most screening is performed in countries with a relatively low incidence of the disease, whereas most women at higher risk of this cancer live in third world countries which do not have extensive screening programmes. When considering the possibility of introducing cervical cancer screening more extensively in a third world country, the lower life expectancy and different age distribution of the population should be taken into account. Also, when considering a screening programme for a population defined other than by geographical area, such as employees or participants in a particular health insurance scheme, it is possible that the age distribution of the screened women is of major influence on cost-effectiveness.

2.4 Screening quality

Two major aspects of quality of breast cancer screening are sensitivity and specificity of the screening test. A low sensitivity can be thought of as the inability to find smaller tumours which can be found by a screening test of better quality; in which case lead time will be shorter and the probability of benefit from the screening is lower. It may also be caused by randomly missing tumours irrespective of their size. This does not lead to a shorter lead time, at least not at the first screening, therefore the average screen-detected case will experience the same benefit from a first screening as in a situation with good sensitivity, but the probability of obtaining this benefit is smaller.

At repeat screenings, the situation becomes more complicated with both false positive and false negative results. Low specificity (i.e. a high false positive rate) does not lead to a lower probability to benefit from the screening, but to a higher probability to suffer from it. False positive screening outcomes lead to undue anxiety and an increased burden of diagnostic procedures which in turn gives rise to extra costs.

The burden of false positive results is often expressed as the positive predictive value, the probability that a case identified at screening truly is positive. For a screening programme in Germany, we estimated the effect of an increase of 12% in sensitivity to be 10% more life-years gained; while a 10% decrease in positive predictive value is expected to lead to a 3% increase in total social cost of the programme (Warmerdam *et al.*, 1997).

2.5 Screening policy

Screening policy is usually either an organised programme with an invitation scheme defined by the ages at which individuals are invited to be screened (ages at which the programme starts and ends, and the intervals between invitations), or it consists of making screening available, with timing dependent primarily on individual decisions (opportunistic screening).

Figure 2.1 shows one aspect of screening policy which is of great importance for the effect to be expected from breast cancer screening. The mortality reduction in a screening programme strongly increases with the number of screenings offered, but under most models, the effectiveness per screening decreases. Note that the percentage mortality reduction as presented here is much lower than mortality reduction reported from randomised controlled trials of screening, since the figure here is on breast cancer mortality in the total population, while a trial considers only the invited cohort.

A programme screening policy and an opportunistic screening policy which would both lead to the same number of screenings would tend to show the following differences: programme screening will lead to a more even spread of screening over the population, more women being screened, with longer intervals, and with intervals more evenly spread over the ages of high risk for the cancer. If these expectations are correct, a programme leads to higher effectiveness per screening than an opportunistic approach.

Because detection rates at first screening tend to be higher than at repeat screenings, the introduction of screening in a population can lead to a temporary increase of cancer

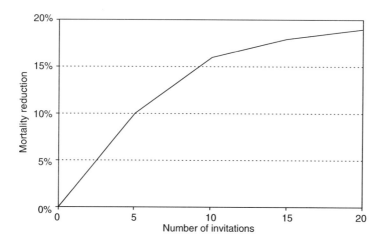

Figure 2.1 Expected mortality reduction from the Dutch national breast cancer screening programme when assuming 70% attendance by the number of invitations issued to the age range of 50–69

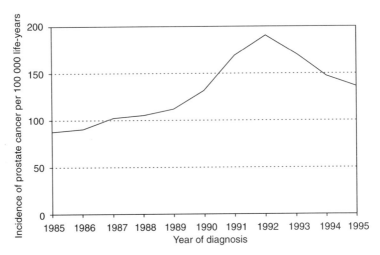

Figure 2.2 Age-adjusted incidence of prostate cancer in the American SEER population by year of diagnosis (Ries *et al.*, 1998)

incidence. A spectacular example of this was observed for prostate cancer by the SEER registry in the USA (Ries *et al.*, 1998). Around the year 1992 there was a sharp peak in prostate cancer incidence (see Figure 2.2). This was contemporaneous with the introduction of prostate specific antigen (PSA) screening, over a relatively short period of time, in the US population. Such rapid introduction would lead to a sharp increase in age-adjusted incidence. After the period of introduction in the population, most men only receive repeat screenings, and the incidence is observed to decrease again. This doubling of new cases of cancer of course led to a major impact on the demand for health care facilities, in this case mainly prostatectomies.

In breast cancer, a similar phenomenon can be observed. The effect will be not as spectacular in mammographic screening for breast cancer, because the prevalence/incidence ratio at first screenings is much lower than in PSA screening. Nevertheless, around the introduction of the breast cancer screening programme in the Netherlands, there was concern firstly as to whether the increase in absolute numbers of new cases of breast cancer would lead to problems with the capacity of radiotherapy, and secondly because early detected breast cancer can often be treated by lumpectomy with radiotherapy instead of mastectomy without radiotherapy for cases diagnosed later in their development. Figure 2.3 shows that the gradual introduction of the national screening programme led to a gradual increase in the demand for radiotherapy, while an instantaneous introduction of the screening programme to all women in the invitation schedule would have led to a much sharper peak in the demand for radiotherapy.

2.6 Screening history

Until recently, there was usually no need for an evaluation study of breast cancer screening in a Western European setting to take into account that there had previously been a significant amount of screening prior to formal introduction of the programme. The first

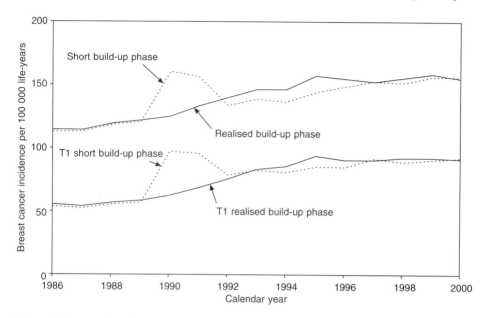

Figure 2.3 Expected incidence in the Dutch population of all breast cancer and of cases of T1 breast cancer as expected with the realised build-up of the national breast screening programme and with an immediate introduction of the programme to all of the target population

report on previous screening influencing a new screening programme was from Bouches du Rhone in France, where it appeared that the programme did not lead to a further improvement in the stage distribution of breast cancer relative to the situation before the official programme, when a substantial amount of opportunistic screening was already taking place (McCann *et al.*, 1997).

Contrary to breast cancer screening, in Western Europe there is a much more extensive history of opportunistic Pap smear screening for the prevention and early detection of cervical cancer and hence the prevention of cervical cancer mortality. Previous screening practice can influence the optimum of a future screening programme in several ways, making it necessary to take this history into account:

- The screening programme will in part be a substitution of the existing practice, leading to fewer effects than would have been observed had the programme been applied to a totally unscreened population. Reduction of incidence and mortality in the population due to the introduction of the programme will be less than the overall effect of screening. Also, the effects on demand for health care facilities will be less salient.
- The age distribution of the screening history may have been far from optimal. For instance in cervical cancer screening, opportunistic screening tends to concentrate in younger ages where most preinvasive lesions are detected, instead of the middle and older ages in which most preventable cancer incidence and mortality occur. This may lead to the conclusion that, particularly at the start of the new programme, an extra effort needs to be made for sufficient screening of middle aged and older women.

2.7 Screening attendance

In breast cancer screening, usually the cost of inviting people to a screening programme is low relative to the cost of the screening procedure as a whole, therefore the cost-effectiveness ratio depends little on attendance. This will be very different for screening for colorectal cancer by a simple faecal occult blood test, for which the cost of performing a screening test is not very different from that of sending out an invitation.

There is a tendency for healthy people and/or people with generally healthy behaviour to be more likely to attend a screening programme than others. In the pilot project on breast cancer screening in Nijmegen (Otten *et al.*, 1996; Verbeek *et al.*, 1984), it was observed that among women aged 68–74, there was a major difference in mortality from other causes than breast cancer between those women attending screening and those not attending, particularly in a short period after the invitation for screening. Women of around age 70 who attended screening had a two-year longer life expectancy than those who did not attend, even without taking into account that the screening may prevent breast cancer death. This means that screening can appear to gain more life-years in older women than would be expected without such a selection effect.

In cervical cancer screening, another selection effect is observed: women attending screening have a lower risk of cervical cancer and its precursors than other women, even if there were no screening effect. That means that the estimated impact on mortality and incidence of cervical cancer in the total population will be markedly less than expected without such a selection effect. Let us consider an example. If attending screening leads to a 90% reduction of cervical cancer mortality, then in a population where 80% of the women attend with no association of attendance with risk, mortality will fall by 80% × 90% = 72%. But if there is a 10% stratum of women who do not attend screening and who have a risk three times higher than other women, then mortality will only go down by $(90\%/(3 \times 10\% + 90\%)) \times 80\% = 60\%$.

2.8 Clinical practice

Diagnostic procedures in women with breast cancer are not likely to vary substantially among screening contexts in Europe: a breast cancer is diagnosed by a biopsy after a number of procedures involving markedly less burden on the woman and on health care costs. For cervical cancer screening the practice of coming to a conclusive diagnosis may be more variable, but will probably still not lead to major differences in cost-effectiveness of cervical screening.

Due to variability of specificity, differences can be greater when seen with respect to diagnostic activity in women without cancer. Low specificity leads to more diagnostic procedures induced by screening. The practice of diagnostics per false positive case can also lead to more or less invasive diagnostic procedures. On the other hand, it is to be expected that screening will reduce diagnostic activity outside screening and this effect can also vary considerably among screening environments.

In cervical cancer screening, variation of diagnostic practice is concentrated in the so-called 'borderline lesions'. The threshold for which cytological abnormalities are regarded as needing further follow-up, and which are not, may vary strongly from one cytological laboratory to the other, and this threshold may vary strongly over time. It is difficult to assess the effects of such differences because new thresholds are not based on randomised trials for their effects on cervical cancer incidence and it is not easy to derive these effects from observational data. Also therapeutic practice may vary among screening contexts and may have a different dependency on stage at detection. For instance in cervical cancer the hysterectomy rate in preinvasive conditions may vary strongly between regions (van Ballegooijen *et al.*, 1995).

2.9 Survival

Survival depends on stage at detection (by screening or clinically) and on the quality of therapy. It is thought that among situations in which cancer screening is considered, variation in survival due to quality of therapy is small in comparison with variation due to stage at detection (Schrijvers *et al.*, 1995). If quality of therapy were to lead to important variations in survival, the effect in general is analogous to that of stage distribution: a more favourable survival leads to less potential effectiveness. However when therapy is not optimal, it is at least possible that treatment of early cases may be particularly unfavourable in comparison with optimal treatment; in that case the improvement of prognosis due to early detection decreases, and thus also the effectiveness of screening.

2.10 Costs

Relevant costs are not only the cost of screening itself, but also of all relevant diagnostic and therapeutic procedures. Medical costs of the life-years saved may also be considered (Drummond *et al.*, 1987; Siegel *et al.*, 1996; Weinstein *et al.*, 1996; Russell *et al.*, 1996). In the evaluation of different breast cancer screening situations up to now, the cost factor which is of greatest influence on cost-effectiveness is whether screening is performed by specialised screening units with an intensive use of the mammographic facilities or as part of a general radiology practice with a relatively low intensity of use of the facilities (van Ineveld *et al.*, 1993).

The unit costs of relevant diagnostic and therapeutic procedures which may vary most strongly between screening situations are those of diagnostics after a positive screening test and of advanced disease. The cost of diagnoses after positive screening tests strongly increases with poorer specificity. The cost of advanced disease as influenced by screening is on the one hand proportional to the number of cancer deaths prevented, therefore also roughly proportional to effectiveness. On the other hand, this cost depends on the amount of medical care a woman with advanced disease receives. This cost per patient is shown to be largely dependent on the average number of hospital days per patient with advanced disease (van Ballegooijen *et al.*, 1992b; Richards *et al.*, 1993; de Koning *et al.*, 1994).

2.11 Balance of favourable and unfavourable health effects

After considering all influences on the effects of cancer screening and trying to quantify them as far as reasonably possible, there comes a time to balance these to make a decision. No cancer screening effort is free of unfavourable effects, therefore the first question to be addressed in making up a balance should be: are the favourable effects outweighing the unfavourable effects? There may be occasions when the answer to this question is obvious. However even in breast cancer screening where the positive effects are well established, this question can become highly relevant when considering different policy alternatives.

An example is defining the best upper age boundary for the invitation schedule of a breast cancer screening programme. Although the incidence and hence the potential benefit of breast cancer increases with age, so does the probability of death from other causes. The latter includes deaths in those with occult breast cancer who would never have incurred the burden of personal anxiety and diagnostic and therapeutic costs had screening not detected their cancers before death from other causes. The strong increase in such negative effects with age means that at some age, the balance of positive and negative effects as expressed by quality adjusted life-years (QALYs) gained by screening becomes so unfavourable that further extension of a screening programme to higher ages does not further increase QALYs gained. This effect is stronger with longer sojourn times of preclinical cancer (Boer *et al.*, 1995). Figure 2.4 shows that if sojourn time does not further increase after age 65, the upper age limit at which the unfavourable effects are expected to outweigh the favourable effect is high, whereas if the sojourn time continues to increase with age, screening beyond age 80 is not expected to gain any more QALYs.

For cervical cancer, there is no detailed published estimate of the balance of positive and negative health effects of screening, and so we have tried to extrapolate our findings for breast cancer screening to cervical cancer screening. Our tentative estimate suggests that the weight of negative effects of this screening can be quite substantial (van Ballegooijen, 1998).

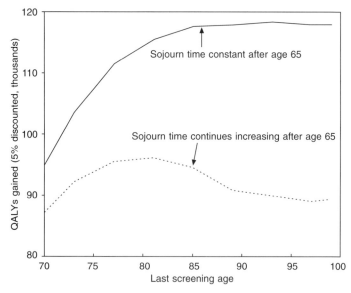

Figure 2.4 Expected number of quality adjusted life-years gained from the Dutch national breast cancer screening programme by upper age limit of a two-yearly screening schedule starting from 50 years old for a model where preclinical screen-detectable sojourn time remains constant from age 65 and for a model where this sojourn time continues to increase

2.12 Time preference

In balancing favourable and unfavourable health effects, as well as effectiveness and costs, for a screening programme, time preference plays an important role. Time preference can be justified by a diversity of theories (Krahn and Gafni, 1993), but they invariably include the notion that benefits of an intervention occurring sooner are considered more favourable than those occurring later. It is customary in cost-effectiveness analysis to express time preference as a yearly discount rate for both health effects and costs, though it has been argued that other models may be better (Cairns and van der Pol, 1997). Because the costs of cancer screening need to be made long before the main targeted effects (prevention of cancer death and possibly incidence) occur, the cost-effectiveness ratio is very sensitive to the applied discount rate. Table 2.3 shows an arbitrary example of cost-effectiveness ratios of cervical cancer screening, illustrating how strongly this ratio depends on discount rate.

Another problem with discounting arises when evaluation of screening concerns a so-called cohort model as opposed to considering a full dynamic population. In the cohort approach it is assumed that all potential participants in a screening programme will be offered the complete invitation schedule and no-one will enter the programme at a later age than the first age of the screening schedule. Applying a discount rate then works out as age preference instead of time preference. This means that screening performed at older ages is assigned an exaggeratedly low weight in the cost-effectiveness ratio as compared to screening at younger ages. To decide which particular ages are to be invited and which not, within an individual programme, this is not a problem, because the marginal cost-effectiveness ratio of adding a screening age to the schedule will be correct. However, in comparisons between programmes, it biases in favour of programmes which derived their cost-effectiveness from younger ages.

2.13 Conclusion

When making prognoses for future new screening programmes, one should obviously begin by interpreting the primary results of trials and observational studies. For extrapolating the results of trials to other screening programmes and other situations, there is a need for more data on background variables such as incidence and stage distribution in the absence of screening. Decisions on whether to initiate a cancer screening programme, and on

Table 2.3 Cost-effectiveness ratios of cervical cancer screening by applied yearly discount rate in a Dutch situation with an invitation policy of seven five-yearly invitations from ages 25–55

Yearly discount rate	Cost effectiveness ratio Dfl/life-year gained
0%	6 248
3%	16 788
5%	29 024
8%	58 399

which screening policy is preferable, should not only depend on the finding that trials show a significant mortality reduction, but should also take several background variables into account. These include epidemiology in the situation without screening, demography, expected screening quality, clinical practice and costs involved.

References

Boer, R., de Koning, H.J., Beemsterboer, P.M., Warmerdam, P.G. and Schroeder, F.H. (1997). A comparison of disease-specific survival of patients who died of and who had newly diagnosed prostate cancer. *J. Urol.*, **157**, 1768–71; discussion 1771–2.

Boer, R., de Koning, H.J., van Oortmarssen, G.J. and van der Maas, P.J. (1995). In search of the best upper age limit for breast cancer screening. *Eur. J. Cancer*, **31A**, 2040–3.

Brown, M.L. and Fintor, L. (1993). Cost-effectiveness of breast cancer screening: preliminary results of a systematic review of the literature. *Breast Cancer Res. Treat.*, **25**, 113–18.

Cairns, J.A. and van der Pol, M.M. (1997). Saving future lives. A comparison of three discounting models. *Health Econ.*, **6**, 341–50.

de Koning, H.J., van Ineveld, B.M., van Oortmarssen, G.J., de Haes, J.C., Collette, H.J., Hendriks, J.H. and van der Maas, P.J. (1991). Breast cancer screening and cost-effectiveness; policy alternatives, quality of life considerations and the possible impact of uncertain factors. *Int. J. Cancer*, **49**, 531–7.

de Koning, H.J., van Dongen, J.A. and van der Maas, P.J. (1994). Changes in use of breast-conserving therapy in years 1978–2000. *Br. J. Cancer*, **70**, 1165–70.

de Koning, H.J., Boer, R., Warmerdam, P.G., Beemsterboer, P.M. and van der Maas, P.J. (1995). Quantitative interpretation of age-specific mortality reductions from the Swedish breast cancer-screening trials. *J. Natl. Cancer Inst.*, **87**, 1217–23.

Drummond, M.F., Stoddart, G.L. and Torrance, G.W. (1987). *Methods for the Economic Evaluation of Health Care Programmes*. Oxford University Press.

Elwood, J.M., Cox, B. and Richardson, A.K. (1993). The effectiveness of breast cancer screening by mammography in younger women. *Online J. Curr. Clin. Trials.*, *32*.

Gustafsson, L., Ponten, J., Bergstrom, R. and Adami, H.O. (1997). International incidence rates of invasive cervical cancer before cytological screening. *Int. J. Cancer*, **71**, 159–65.

Habbema, J.D., van Oortmarssen, G.J., Lubbe, J.T. and van der Maas, P.J. (1985). The MISCAN simulation program for the evaluation of screening for disease. *Comput. Methods Programs Biomed.*, **20**, 79–93.

Koopmanschap, M.A., van Oortmarssen, G.J., van Agt, H.M., van Ballegooijen, M., Habbema, J.D. and Lubbe, K.T. (1990). Cervical-cancer screening: attendance and cost-effectiveness. *Int. J. Cancer*, **45**, 410–15.

Krahn, M. and Gafni, A. (1993). Discounting in the economic evaluation of health care interventions. *Med. Care*, **31**, 403–18.

Loeve, F., Boer, R., Oortmarssen, G.J., van Ballegooijen, M. and Habbema, J.D.F. (1999). The MISCAN-COLON simulation model for the evaluation of colorectal cancer screening. *Comput. Biomed. Res.*, **32**, 13–33.

McCann, J., Wait, S., Seradour, B. and Day, N. (1997). A comparison of the performance and impact of breast cancer screening programmes in East Anglia, UK and Bouches du Rhone, France. *Eur. J. Cancer*, **33**, 429–35.

Otten, J.D., van Dijck, J.A., Peer, P.G., Straatman, H., Verbeek, A.L., Mravunac, M., Hendriks, J.H. and Holland, R. (1996). Long term breast cancer screening in Nijmegen, the Netherlands: the nine rounds from 1975–92. *J. Epidemiol. Community Health*, **50**, 353–8.

Paci, E., Boer, R., Zappa, M., de Koning, H.J., van Oortmarssen, G.J., Crocetti, E., Giorgi, D., Rosselli del Turco, M. and Habbema, J.D. (1995). A model-based prediction of the impact on reduction in mortality by a breast cancer screening programme in the city of Florence, Italy. *Eur. J. Cancer*, **31A**, 348–53.

Richards, M.A., Braysher, S., Gregory, W.M. and Rubens, R.D. (1993). Advanced breast cancer: use of resources and cost implications. *Br. J. Cancer*, **67**, 856–60.

Ries, L.A.G., Kosary, C.L., Hankey, B.F., Miller, B.A. and Edwards, B.K. (1998). *SEER Cancer Statistics Review, 1973–1995*. National Cancer Institute, Bethesda, MD.

Russell, L.B., Gold, M.R., Siegel, J.E., Daniels, N. and Weinstein, M.C. (1996). The role of cost-effectiveness analysis in health and medicine. *JAMA*, **276**, 1172–7.

Schrijvers, T.M., Coebergh, J.-W.W., van der Heijden, L.H. and Mackenbach, J.P. (1995). Socioeconomic variation in cancer survival in the Southeastern Netherlands. *Cancer*, **75**, 2946–53.

Siegel, J.E., Weinstein, M.C., Russell, L.B. and Gold, M.R. (1996). Recommendations for reporting cost-effectiveness analyses. *JAMA*, **276**, 1339–41.

van Ballegooijen, M. (1998). Effects and costs of cervical cancer screening. Thesis, iMGZ, Rotterdam.

van Ballegooijen, M., Koopmanschap, M.A., van Oortmarssen, G.J., Habbema, J.D., Lubbe, K.T. and van Agt, H.M. (1990). Diagnostic and treatment procedures induced by cervical cancer screening. *Eur. J. Cancer*, **26**, 941–5.

van Ballegooijen, M., Habbema, J.D., van Oortmarssen, G.J., Koopmanschap, M.A., Lubbe, J.T. and van Agt, H.M. (1992a). Preventive Pap-smears: balancing costs, risks and benefits. *Br. J. Cancer*, **65**, 930–3.

van Ballegooijen, M., Koopmanschap, M.A., Tjokrowardojo, A.J. and van Oortmarssen, G.J. (1992b). Care and costs for advanced cervical cancer. *Eur. J. Cancer*, **28A**, 1703–8.

van Ballegooijen, M., Koopmanschap, M.A. and Habbema, J.D. (1995). The management of cervical intraepithelial neoplasia (CIN): extensiveness and costs in The Netherlands. *Eur. J. Cancer*, **10**, 1672–6.

van Ballegooijen, M., van den Akker-van Marle, M.E., Warmerdam, P.G., Meijer, C.J., Walboomers, J.M. and Habbema, J.D. (1997). Present evidence on the value of HPV testing for cervical cancer screening: a model-based exploration of the (cost-) effectiveness. *Br. J. Cancer*, **76**, 651–7.

van Ineveld, B.M., van Oortmarssen, G.J., de Koning, H.J., Boer, R. and van der Maas, P.J. (1993). How cost-effective is breast cancer screening in different EC countries? *Eur. J. Cancer*, **12**, 1663–8.

van Oortmarssen, G.J., Habbema, J.D., van der Maas, P.J., de Koning, H.J., Collette, H.J., Verbeek, A.L., Geerts, A.T. and Lubbe, K.T. (1990). A model for breast cancer screening. *Cancer*, **66**, 1601–12.

Verbeek, A.L., Hendriks, J.H., Holland, R., Mravunac, M., Sturmans, F. and Day, N.E. (1984). Reduction of breast cancer screening mortality through mass screening with modern mammography. First results of the Nijmegen project, 1975–1981. *Lancet*, **1**, 1222–4.

Warmerdam, P.G., Koning, H.J., de Boer, R., Beemsterboer, P.M.M., Dierks, M.-L., Swart, E. and Robra, B.-P. (1997). Quantitative estimates of the impact of sensitivity and specificity in mammographic screening in Germany. *J. Epidemiol. Community Health*, **51**, 180–6.

Weinstein, M.C., Siegel, J.E., Gold, M.R., Kamlet, M.S. and Russell, L.B. (1996). Recommendations of the Panel on Cost-effectiveness in Health and Medicine. *JAMA*, **276**, 1253–8.

3

Contamination and non-compliance in screening trials

Jack Cuzick

3.1 Departures from screening trial protocol

Failure to comply with the allocated treatment is a major problem in randomised screening trials and can lead to a considerable decay in the power available to detect any real benefits from screening. Arguably, in a trial of a preventive intervention in healthy subjects, there is less incentive for the study subjects to comply with protocol than in a therapeutic trial on individuals with disease. The power loss from non-compliance is proportional to the square of the percentage of compliant patients so that, for example, if this is 70%, the trial needs to be twice as large to achieve the same power as that obtained for perfect compliance. This factor becomes 4-fold for 50% compliance and 10-fold for 30% compliance.

Two distinct but theoretically similar problems arise when dealing with differences between allocated and actual treatment, depending on the arm to which an individual is allocated. They are referred to as non-compliance and contamination.

3.2 Non-compliance

Non-compliance refers to the situation in which an individual allocated to screening refuses to accept this opportunity. This can be a particularly difficult problem for new approaches to screening that are invasive or unpleasant. A good example is colorectal cancer screening. Two methodologies are potentially beneficial but both carry social taboos or a degree of unpleasantness. Faecal occult blood testing is relatively simple, but suffers from inhibitions about anything to do with bowels, and because it must be done every 1–2 years, compliance must be maintained for several years. Once-off compliance rates have ranged from 20–75% (Verne *et al.*, 1998; Hardcastle *et al.*, 1996; Petrelli *et al.*, 1994; Kronborg *et al.*, 1996; Mandel *et al.*, 1993). Sigmoidoscopy is a more invasive procedure, also loaded with social taboos, but only needs to be performed once in a lifetime, or very infrequently. Compliance rates of 30–40% have been reported in some studies (Verne *et al.*, 1998; Atkin *et al.*, 1998), but have been as low as 20% (Berry *et al.*, 1997).

Compliance can be more difficult at the trial stage than for a service screening programme, because at the former stage public education and propaganda cannot ethically be offered. Once a test has been shown to be efficacious, such as for cervical screening, large-scale education about its benefits can be undertaken, but this is improper at the stage of evaluation, so that the compliance achievable in a programme can be much higher than for a trial.

One approach that can artificially improve compliance within a trial is to send a prerandomisation questionnaire to all prospective entrants, and to only randomise those who express some willingness to be screened if it is offered. It is still crucial that randomisation is actually performed so that like is compared with like. It is not appropriate to offer screening only to those that are interested, and compare them to those that are not interested, as this can lead to a serious bias. This prerandomisation questionnaire approach has been used in a large trial of once in a lifetime sigmoidscopy in the United Kingdom to good effect. Eligible individuals, aged 55–64, were sent a letter advising them of the health services' interest in offering colorectal screening, and were given a short description of the test, and the potential risks and benefits. They were then asked 'If you were invited to have the bowel cancer screening test, would you take up the offer?' They would answer either 'Definitely YES, Probably YES, Probably NO, or Definitely NOT'. About 60% of these approached replied in the former two categories and only those were randomised into the trial. Only individuals allocated treatment (one-third of those randomised) were then approached again. This was done via a personal letter from their general practitioner, which is also very important, and a more detailed information pack was included. A 70% compliance has been achieved (Atkin *et al.*, 1998), compared to the 30–40% likely if standard procedures had been used, leading to adequate power with a trial of one-third the size that would have been required otherwise.

Five things appear to be important for good compliance:

1. good information materials;
2. a personal letter from the patient's own general practitioner (even if scanned signatures and letterheads are used);
3. flexible scheduling;
4. excellent screening procedures and backup support; and
5. selection of a population likely to be compliant.

The last of these raises questions of generalisability. It is a reasonable assumption that the *relative* benefits of screening are likely to be similar in a health conscious subpopulation, but the baseline risks may well be different, and the compliance rates will certainly be different. The two latter issues become very important for a screening programme, once a modality is accepted as efficacious, but these are very much second-stage questions. The primary goal of a trial should be to evaluate efficacy accurately. This is typically the most difficult issue, and it can be seriously undermined if concerns about other aspects lead to an increased failure of individuals to accept their allocated treatment.

3.3 Contamination

Contamination is the reverse type of non-compliance in which control individuals actively seek out the experimental treatment. It can also have severe effects, especially when the screening procedure under consideration is generally available and propaganda exists to suggest that it is effective. This is a serious problem for evaluating prostate specific antigen testing for prostate cancer, or mammography for breast cancer screening in younger women (aged < 50), especially in the United States. This was a problem even for evaluating the older trials of chest X-ray screening for lung cancer, which were done at a time when this was generally perceived as being efficacious. The net detrimental effect on power is similar to non-compliance, in that the effective sample size is reduced by the square of the non-contaminant percentage. When both non-compliance and contamination are present, the effects can be extremely severe, as each effect percentage must be subtracted from 100% before squaring to get the effective sample size. Thus even a 20% non-compliance rate coupled with a 10% contamination can lead to a 50% reduction in effective sample size and a 30% non-compliance combined with a 20% contamination rate will lead to a 4-fold reduction to the effective sample size.

Delayed contamination can also be a problem for screening trials, where prolonged follow-up is the norm. This is particularly troublesome when preliminary information, often from other studies, suggests that screening may be beneficial. This can lead to members of the control population subsequently deciding to request screening, or in some cases even being offered it. This is a potential weakness in designs that focus on health conscious individuals, as considered above. Selection of a population of good compliers is likely to increase the risk of contamination, and the two aspects of non-compliance and contamination need to be balanced in a way to maximise the number of 'uncommitted' individuals who are randomised. Delayed non-compliance can also be a problem for screening modalities that require periodic testing.

3.4 Adjusting for non-compliance and contamination

A direct comparison of those receiving screening with those who did not can lead to serious biases, since individuals who avail themselves of screening tests are often healthier and have different baseline risks than those who do not. This is an important problem in the analysis and interpretation of case-control studies and underscores the importance of randomisation, as a way of comparing like with like. However, the conventional intention-to-treat analysis poses problems for randomised comparisons, as non-compliance can lead to diluted treatment differences. Such an analysis gives an estimate of the effect of an intervention on the entire population offered screening, assuming that compliance rates will be the same in a large-scale screening programme as they were in the trial. In many cases it is of greater interest to know the effect of the intervention among those who comply. Consideration of how to improve compliance in a population-wide programme then becomes a separate issue. Indeed, compliance within a trial does not necessarily reflect that which is achievable within a programme, where it can be better or worse, depending on the available infrastructure and the extent of a public education programme.

A naive comparison of those screened versus those not screened is beset by the same biases as case-control studies, and cannot be recommended. However, recently methods have been developed which allow an unbiased assessment of the effectiveness of the intervention in those who actually receive it, but which still fully respects the randomisation. Building on ideas of Sommer and Zeger (1991), Cuzick *et al.* (1997) have developed a method which will adjust for both non-compliance and contamination in studies with binomial outcomes, for example where the outcome of interest is death from or occurrence of the disease in question or not, with no consideration of time to death or occurrence. This model is generally appropriate for screening trials, since the proportion of individuals destined to develop disease is small, so that there is little to be gained in accounting for the time at which disease occurs (Cuzick, 1982).

The general scheme is outlined in Figure 3.1. The population is split into three latent groups: (i) insistors who will demand the treatment whether randomised to it or not; (ii) refusers, who will not take the treatment even if offered; and (iii) the ambivalent remainder who will accept what is offered. These three groups are not fully observed, but randomisation guarantees that they will be split into those allocated to treatment and control in the same proportions, on average. In particular, refusers are only directly identified in the treatment arm, whereas insistors are identified only in the control arm; the remaining groups are mixed. However, potential refusers and insistors in the mixed groups can be inferred from the corresponding group in the other arm of the trial. The following example illustrates our approach (see Figure 3.2).

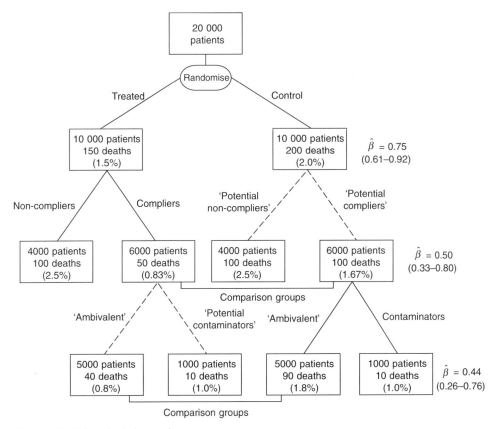

Figure 3.1 A hypothetical example

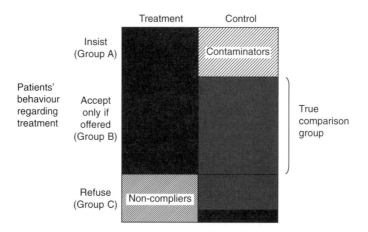

Figure 3.2 Schematic representation of the three types of patients and two treatment options. Failure rates can only be observed in the four shaded groups, and true treatment differences in the ambivalent populations must be inferred

Consider a trial of 20 000 patients who are randomised equally to treatment or control, and who are followed up for a similar length of time. Assume 200 deaths occur in the control arm (2%) and 150 occur in the treated arm (1.5%). Then an intent-to-treat analysis would show a 25% reduction in the death rate ($p = 0.006$) with a 95% confidence interval of (8–39%). However, further investigation showed that 100 of the deaths in the treated group occurred in 4000 patients who refused the treatment, so that the death rate in the 6000 treated patients was only 0.83% (50/6000). The apparent reduction compared to the control group is now 58%, but this is a biased estimate because the rate in the refusers was 2.5% which is higher than for controls. However, if one uses the rate for refusers in the treated group as a surrogate for the comparable subgroup amongst controls, we would infer that 4000 controls would be latent refusers, and among these 100 deaths would be expected. The remaining 6000 controls would have experienced the remaining 100 deaths for a death rate of 1.67%. This is the appropriate group to compare compliers against and yields a reduction of 50% $\left(100\% - \dfrac{50/6000}{100/6000}\right)$.

To take this further, assume that 1000 of the controls actively sought and obtained the treatment and there were 10 deaths in the group (1%). By randomisation there was a comparable group in the group allocated treatment who on average would have fared similarly. If we subtract out this group as well, we are left with 40 deaths in the 5000 patients randomised to treatment who complied but who were estimated to not have sought treatment if not invited. This group has a death rate of 0.8%. If this is compared to the estimated 90 deaths in the 5000 controls who did not have the treatment, but were estimated to accept it if offered, the estimated reduction in death rate is 56% $\left(100\% - \dfrac{40/5000}{90/5000}\right)$. The confidence intervals in Figure 3.1 can be computed by the methods indicated in Cuzick *et al.* (1997).

3.5 Adjusting for covariates

The methods used to obtain these estimates are developed and described in detail by Cuzick et al. (1997). In that paper, no individual covariates were considered, and here we show how to extend that analysis to the situation in which covariates are also allowed.

At first sight, one might be confused as to the need for adjustment for covariates in the context of a randomised trial, since the randomisation should balance covariate patterns on average between the study and control groups. However, it is possible that chance variation between the groups, for example with respect to age, may cause some inaccuracy in the estimated treatment effect, despite being compatible with random allocation. In addition, non-compliance or contamination may itself be partly confounded with age or other covariates. It may therefore be of use to adjust for covariates in some cases.

We use an underlying logistic model and the following notation. Let γ_k ($k = 1, 2, 3$) be the log-odds ratios for disease in insistors, ambivalents and refusers, respectively. Let β_0 be the log-odds ratio for a screening benefit, z_0 be the indicator function for allocated to treatment, and $z_i^* = (z_{1i}, z_{2i}, ..., z_{mi})^T$ be the individual covariates with regression coefficients $\beta^* = (\beta_1, \beta_2, ..., \beta_m)^T$. Let $\beta = (\beta_0, \beta^{*T})^T$, $z_i = (z_{i0}, z_i^{*T})^T$ and let α_k ($k = 1, 2, 3$) denote the (observed) proportions of control insistors, ambivalents and refusers (allocated treatment), respectively. If

$$(w_1, w_2, w_3) = \begin{cases} (1, 0, 0), & \text{control – insistor} \\ (0, 1, 1), & \text{control – untreated} \\ (1, 1, 0), & \text{treatment – accepts} \\ (0, 0, 1), & \text{treatment – refuses} \end{cases}$$

are used to reflect into which of the four observed groups an individual falls, and δ_i indicates that individual i developed the disease in question, the likelihood can be written as follows:

$$L = \prod_i \frac{\sum_{k=1}^{3} \alpha_k w_{ki} \, p(\delta_i, \beta^T z_i + \gamma_k)}{\sum_{k=1}^{3} \alpha_k w_{ki}}$$

where $p(\delta, x) = (e^{\delta x}/(1 + e^x))$ is the usual logistic probability function and w_{ki} are the components (w_1, w_2, w_3) for the ith individual. When no individual covariates exist, this reduces to four parameters ($\gamma_1, \gamma_2, \gamma_3, \beta_0$) which can be estimated uniquely from the four observed groups. The relative risk parameter studied in Cuzick et al. (1997) can be identified as

$$e^{\beta_0} \left(\frac{1 + e^{\gamma_2}}{1 + e^{\gamma_2 + \beta_0}} \right)$$

In the more general set-up we can form score equations and an information matrix in the usual way, using the first and second derivatives of the likelihood function. For mathematical readers, the score equations are shown in the appendix.

References

Atkin, W.S., Hart, A., Edwards, R., McIntyre, P., Aubrey, R., Wardle, J., Sutton, S., Cuzick, J. and Northover, J.M.A. (1998). Uptake, yield of neoplasia, and adverse effects on flexible sigmoidoscopy screening. *Gut*, **42**, 560–5.

Berry, D.P., Clarke, P., Hardcastle, J.D. and Vellacott, K.D. (1997). Randomized trial of the addition of flexible sigmoidoscopy to faecal occult blood testing for colorectal neoplasia population screening. *British Journal of Surgery*, **84**, 1274–6.

Cuzick, J. (1982). The efficiency of the proportions test and the logrank test for censored survival data. *Biometrics*, **38**, 1033–9.

Cuzick, J., Edwards, R. and Segnan, N. (1997). Adjusting for non-compliance and contamination in randomized clinical trials. *Statistics in Medicine*, **16**, 1017–29.

Hardcastle, J.D., Chamberlain, J.O., Robinson, M.H.E., Moss, S.M., Amar, S.S., Balfour, T.W., James, P.D. and Mangham, C.M. (1996). Randomised controlled trial of faecal-occult-blood screening for colorectal cancer. *Lancet*, **348**, 1472–7.

Kronborg, O., Fenger, C., Olsen, J., Jørgensen, O.D. and Søndergaard, O. (1996). Randomised study of screening for colorectal cancer with faecal-occult-blood test. *Lancet*, **348**, 1467–71.

Mandel, J.S., Bond, J.H., Church, T.R., Snover, D.C., Bradley, M., Schuman, L.M. and Ederer, F. (1993). Reducing mortality from colorectal cancer by screening for fecal occult blood. *New England Journal of Medicine*, **328**, 1365–71.

Petrelli, N., Michalek, A.M., Freedman, A., Baroni, M., Mink, I. and Rodriguez-Bigs, M. (1994). Immunochemical versus guaiac occult blood stool tests: results of a community-based screening program. *Surgical Oncology*, **3**, 27–36.

Sommer, A. and Zeger, S.L. (1991). On estimating efficacy from clinical trials. *Statistics in Medicine*, **10**, 45–52.

Verne, J.E., Aubrey, R., Love, S.B., Talbot, I.C. and Northover, J.M. (1998). Population based randomised study of uptake and yield of screening by flexible sigmoidoscopy compared with screening by faecal occult blood testing. *BMJ*, **317**, 182–5.

Appendix: Score equations for estimation in the presence of covariates

We create a new vector $z_{ik} = (z_i, v_{1k}, n_{2k}, n_{3k})$, where $v_{lk} = \delta_{lk}$ is Kronecker's delta, so that there are indicators for individual i being an insistor, ambivalent, or refuser respectively, as $k = 1, 2, 3$, so that each individual now contributes three terms. Now augment $\beta = (\beta_0, \ldots, \beta_{m+3})$ where $\beta_{m+k} = \gamma_k$, $k = 1, 2, 3$; and write $\alpha_{ki} = \alpha_k w_{ki}$ so that

$$\frac{d \log L}{d\beta} = \sum_i \frac{\displaystyle\sum_{k=1}^{3} \alpha_{ki} p_{ki} \frac{d \log p(\delta_i, \beta^{\mathrm{T}} z_{ik})}{d\beta}}{\displaystyle\sum_k \alpha_{ki} p_{ki}}$$

where $p_{ki} = p(1, \beta^{\mathrm{T}} z_{ik})$; and

$$\frac{d^2 \log L}{d\beta d\beta^{\mathrm{T}}} = \sum_i \frac{\displaystyle\sum_{k=1}^{3} \alpha_{ki} p_{ki} \frac{d^2 \log p(\delta_i, \beta^{\mathrm{T}} z_{ik})}{d\beta d\beta^{\mathrm{T}}}}{\displaystyle\sum_k \alpha_{ki} p_{ki}}$$

$$+ \sum_i \frac{\displaystyle\sum_{k=1}^{3} \alpha_{ki} p_{ki} \left\{ \frac{d \log p(\delta_i, \beta^{\mathrm{T}} z_{ik})}{d\beta} \right\}^{\otimes 2}}{\displaystyle\sum_k \alpha_{ki} p_{ki}}$$

$$- \sum_i \frac{\left\{ \displaystyle\sum_{k=1}^{3} \alpha_{ki} p_{ki} \frac{d \log p(\delta_i, \beta^{\mathrm{T}} z_{ik})}{d\beta} \right\}^{\otimes 2}}{\left(\displaystyle\sum_k \alpha_{ki} p_{ki} \right)^2}$$

where $\otimes 2$ denotes the outer product, e.g. $z^{\otimes 2} = z z^{\mathrm{T}}$.

Here, as usual

$$\frac{d \log p(\delta_i, \beta^{\mathrm{T}} z_{ik})}{d\beta} = z(\delta_i - p_{ki})$$

and

$$\frac{d^2 \log p(\delta_i, \beta^{\mathrm{T}} z_{ik})}{d\beta d\beta^{\mathrm{T}}} = -z z^{\mathrm{T}} (p_{ki} - p_{ki}^2)$$

Estimation and asymptotic analysis can be carried out from these equations in a standard fashion by iterative solution for β. Since the likelihoods are mixtures of log-concave likelihoods, convergence to a unique solution is always guaranteed. For small samples the log-likelihoods can be highly non-quadratic and use of the profile likelihood directly for confidence interval estimation is recommended (see Cuzick et al., 1997).

4

Evaluating periodic cancer screening without a randomised control group: a simplified design and analysis

Stuart G. Baker

4.1 Introduction

The main difficulty with evaluating cancer screening without a randomised control group is the strong possibility of selection bias: subjects who receive screening generally differ from those who do not in terms of factors affecting cancer incidence and possibly cancer mortality. Periodic Screening Evaluation (PSE) is a special design and analysis which can reduce selection bias when there are no randomised controls. PSE estimates the reduction in cancer mortality due to starting periodic cancer screening at a younger age. The key idea is to use older screened subjects as controls for younger screened subjects when estimating age-specific incidence in the absence of a control group. Although special assumptions are required, we believe they are reasonable for some types of cancer screening. PSE was formulated by Baker (1989) and Baker and Chu (1990) and subsequently refined in Baker (1998). This article presents a simplified design and analysis.

4.2 Study design

Suppose investigators wish to evaluate periodic cancer screening at intervals of one year starting at age 40 versus age 60. (One could substitute any length interval or age range.) For PSE, investigators need to invite subjects aged 40–60 to two screens one year apart. Some subjects will refuse and some will accept the screening invitation. Determining cancer mortality rates requires long-term follow-up of acceptors detected with cancer on screening or in the interval between screenings and for refusers detected with cancer within one year of the start of the study. A sample size formula is given in Section 4.8.

4.3 Assumptions

For PSE to give a valid estimate of the effect of screening on cancer mortality, the following assumptions must hold:

Assumption 1: Once screening is positive it will always be positive. We say screening is positive if the screening test is positive and it is confirmed by biopsy.
Assumption 2: Given age, the probability of cancer detection does not depend on year of birth.
Assumption 3: Cancer mortality rates following detection of cancer due to symptoms are the same in refusers as in subjects who received screening, had they not been screened.

Assumption 1 most likely holds when non-microscopic tumours are required for detection on biopsy. Assumption 1 implies a continuous period of time up to detection resulting from symptoms when cancer can be detected on screening and confirmed by biopsy. Assumption 1 does not preclude false negative screening tests (the test is negative but a biopsy would have found cancer) or false positive screening tests (the test is positive and biopsy does not find cancer); these can occur prior to the period of when both the screening test and biopsy would be positive.

   Assumption 2 is implicit whenever the results of a screening study are extrapolated to the future. PSE also requires Assumption 2 to hold for past data. Moran (1998) has investigated the bias associated with violations in Assumption 2.

   Assumption 3 says that once a subject is detected with cancer, the time course of the subsequent disease is unrelated to factors affecting the decision to receive screening. Assumption 3 is the least likely to hold *a priori*. However, using data from a randomised control group, Baker (1998) verified that it was reasonable when applied to breast cancer screening in the Health Insurance Plan of Greater New York (HIP) study (Shapiro *et al.*, 1988).

4.4 Estimating age-specific cancer incidence

Suppose data have been collected from the design in Section 4.2 to evaluate yearly periodic cancer screening starting at age 40 versus age 60. The first analytic step is to estimate the age-specific incidence of cancer following various types of detection. Let $a = 40, 41, \ldots, 60$, denote the age of a subject at the start of study. Among asymptomatic subjects scheduled for screens at ages a and $a + 1$, there are three types of cancer detection (Figure 4.1):

$F =$ positive First screening at age a;
$I =$ negative screening at age a and symptomatic cancer in the following one year Interval prior to the screening at age $a + 1$;
$S =$ negative screening at age a, no symptomatic cancer in the following one year interval; and a positive Subsequent screening at age $a + 1$.

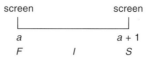

Figure 4.1 Types of cancer detection in the study design for 40, 41, . . . , 59, 60

In the absence of screening, there is one type of cancer detection:

N = symptomatic cancer after no screening in the interval between a and $a + 1$.

Let $q_d(a)$ denote the probability of type d cancer detection associated with age a. For $d = F, I$ and S, the estimated $q_d(a)$ is the number of subjects with type d detection for age a divided by the number of subjects at risk. Invoking Assumption 1 gives the key equation for reducing selection bias:

$$q_N(a) = q_F(a) + q_I(a) + q_S(a) - q_F(a + 1) \tag{4.1}$$

where $q_F(a + 1)$ is the probability of a positive first screening at age $a + 1$ after a hypothetical one-year delay from the start of the study. See Appendix A for a proof.

Using data from the study design it is not possible to directly estimate $q_F(a + 1)$ because no subjects are invited to a first screening after a one-year delay. However, by invoking Assumption 2, one can estimate $q_F(a + 1)$ from subjects aged $a + 1$ who are detected on the first screening at the start of the study. Because these subjects are one year older than hypothetical subjects who receive a first screening at age $a + 1$ after a one-year delay, this estimation procedure uses older screened subjects as controls for younger screened subjects.

To illustrate (4.1) suppose 400 subjects aged 40 are invited for screening with two detected on the first screening, one in the interval, and three on the second screening. Also suppose that 800 subjects aged 41 are invited for screening and four are detected on the first screening. Our estimates are $q_F(40) = 2/400$, $q_I(40) = 1/398$, $q_S(40) = 3/397$ and $q_N(40) = 2/400 + 1/398 + 3/397 - 4/800 =$ approximately 4/400.

4.5 Estimating cumulative cancer mortality following detection

The second analytic step computes m_d, the estimated cumulative cancer mortality following type d cancer detection. To adjust for censoring, one should compute m_d as one minus the actuarial survival estimate (Cox and Oakes, 1984). Under Assumption 3, cancer mortality data from refusers is used to estimate m_N.

4.6 Using a surrogate endpoint for cumulative cancer mortality

If screening technology is changing rapidly over time, long-term follow-up may be unacceptable as the results of the study may only apply to obsolete technology. In that case, one could make an additional assumption and use a short-term surrogate endpoint to estimate m_d. As an example, consider a surrogate endpoint s such that $s = 0$ if the lymph

Table 4.1 Five-year cumulative cancer mortality rates given node state and type of detection

Node state	HIP study			BCDDP		
	First screen cancers	Interval cancers	Subsequent screen cancers	First screen cancers	Interval cancers	Subsequent screen cancers
Negative	0.03	0.18	0.04	0.04	0.11	0.04
Positive	0.38	0.55	0.35	0.15	0.33	0.08

nodes are negative for cancer, and $s = 1$ if positive. Using the surrogate endpoint, the estimated cumulative cancer mortality after type d detection is

$$m_d = (1 - w_d)c_{0d} + w_d c_{1d}$$

where w_d is the estimated probability of a positive node given type d detection, and c_{sd} is the estimated cumulative probability of cancer death following node state s on type d detection. To shorten the duration of the study, one uses data from the trial to estimate w_d and data from a previous study to estimate c_{sd}. Let n denote the number of subjects screened in the current study and n^* denote the number screened in a previous study. The expected number with negative nodes in the previous study is n^*w_d; the expected number with positive nodes in the previous study is $n^*(1 - w_d)$. Using the delta method and assuming binomial distributions, the asymptotic variance of m_d is

$$\text{var}(m_d) = \frac{(1 - w_d)^2 c_{0d}(1 - c_{0d})}{n^*(1 - w_d)} + \frac{w_d^2 c_{1d}(1 - c_{1d})}{n^* w_d} + \frac{(1 - w_d)w_d(c_{1d} - c_{0d})}{n}$$

$$(4.2)$$

If c_{sd} is estimated from the current study, $n^* = n$ and (4.2) reduces to the overall binomial variance. In this framework, there is no gain in efficiency with a surrogate endpoint unless n^* is larger than n. The main problem with using surrogate endpoints is the potential for bias. The underlying assumption is that data from a previous study provide a good estimate of c_{sd}. Table 4.1 compares estimates of c_{sd} from two studies of breast cancer screening, the HIP, which took place in the early 1960s, and the Breast Cancer Detection Demonstration Project (BCDDP), which took place in the 1970s.

Estimates for HIP were computed from the raw data and estimates for BCDDP come from Morrison *et al.* (1988). The difference between HIP and BCDDP in the probability of cancer death given positive node may be due to introduction of adjuvant therapies. If one applied the HIP estimates to surrogate endpoints in BCDDP, estimates of the cumulative cancer mortality rates after detection would be substantially biased. Note that this is not the same framework for surrogate endpoints considered by Prentice (1989).

4.7 Estimating the reduction in cancer mortality due to periodic screening

The final step is to combine the age-specific incidences and the cancer mortality rates after detection to estimate the reduction in cancer mortality due to starting periodic

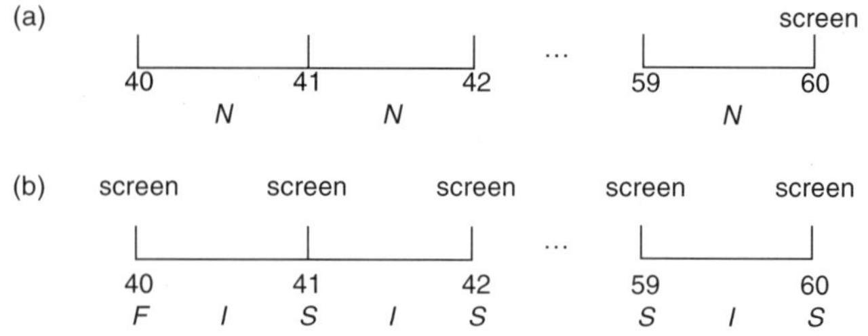

Figure 4.2 Types of cancer detection for evaluating periodic cancer screening starting at age 40 versus age 60

cancer screening at a younger age. Ignoring deaths from competing risks greatly simplifies the formula in Baker (1998). For evaluating breast cancer screening between ages 40 and 60, this simplification had only a small effect on the estimate.

To evaluate periodic cancer screening between ages 40 and 60, let

$$Q_d = \sum_{a=40}^{59} q_d(a)$$

denote the cumulative probability of type d detection between ages 40 and 60. To simplify notation, we define $q_F = q_F(40)$ and $q_{F*} = q_F(60)$. When screening starts at age 60 (Figure 4.2(a)), the cumulative probability of cancer mortality due to cancer detection between ages 40 and 60 is $Q_N m_N + q_{F*} m_F$. When screening starts at age 40 (Figure 4.2(b)), the cumulative probability of cancer mortality due to cancer detection between ages 40 and 60 is $q_F m_F + Q_I m_I + Q_S m_S$. Therefore, the reduction in cancer mortality due to starting screening at age 40 instead of 60 is the difference

$$g = (Q_N m_N + q_{F*} m_F) - (q_F m_F + Q_I m_I + Q_S m_S) \tag{4.3}$$

Substituting (4.1) into (4.3) gives the simple formula

$$g = (q_F - q_{F*})(m_N - m_F) + Q_I(m_N - m_I) + Q_S(m_N - m_S) \tag{4.4}$$

Let v_d denote the variance of m_d computed using Greenwood's formula to account for censoring (e.g. Cox and Oakes, 1984). Assuming a Poisson distribution and using the delta method, the asymptotic variance of g is

$$\text{var}(g) = \left(\frac{q_F}{n(40)} + \frac{q_{F*}}{n(60)} \right)(m_N - m_F)^2 + \sum_{a=40}^{59} \frac{q_I(a)}{n(a)}(m_N - m_I)^2$$

$$+ \sum_{a=40}^{59} \frac{q_S(a)}{n(a)}(m_N - m_S)^2$$

$$+ (q_F - q_{F*})^2 (v_N + v_F) + Q_I^2 (v_N + v_I) + Q_S^2 (v_N + v_S) \tag{4.5}$$

where $n(a)$ is the number aged a at the first screen.

4.8 Sample size

Let θ denote the anticipated reduction in the probability of cancer death. For starting periodic screening at age 40 instead of age 60, the anticipated reduction in cancer mortality is $g = Q_N m_N \theta$, where Q_N is the anticipated cumulative probability of cancer detection between ages 40 and 60 in the absence of screening and m_N is the anticipated cumulative cancer mortality following detection in the absence of screening.

Define $\sigma^2/n = \text{var}(g)$, where $n = n(a)$ is the number of subjects screened per age interval. If π denotes the fraction of subjects expected to refuse screening, the number of subjects offered screening per age interval equals $n/(1 - \pi)$. Therefore, for a two-sided type I error of 0.05 and a power of 0.8, the sample size offered screening is

$$\frac{1}{1 - \pi} \frac{(1.96 + 1.28)^2 \sigma^2}{(Q_N m_N \theta)^2} \tag{4.6}$$

The difficulty with using (4.6) is specifying the parameters in (4.5) which are needed to compute σ^2. As derived in Appendix B, we approximate σ^2 by the following formula involving many fewer parameters:

$$\sigma^2 \approx (\alpha^2 + (1 - \alpha)^2) Q_N \left(\frac{1}{\alpha} + \frac{1 - \pi}{\pi} \right) \Big/ 4 \tag{4.7}$$

where $\alpha = Q_I/Q_N$. To illustrate the calculations, suppose $Q_N = 0.05$, $\alpha = 1/3$, $\pi = 1/3$, $\theta = 0.25$ and $m_N = 0.5$. Applying (4.6) and (4.7) gives a sample size of 14 000 per age interval. Unfortunately, this sample size calculation can sometimes be extremely conservative; more refinements are necessary. When using a surrogate endpoint with data from a previous study of approximately the same size, the same formula would apply.

4.9 Estimating the false positive rate

A balanced evaluation of cancer screening should report the downside of screening as well as any reduction in cancer mortality. Perhaps the primary downside is unnecessary biopsies. See Elmore *et al.* (1998) for a discussion of other downsides to screening. To estimate the number of unnecessary biopsies associated with periodic cancer screening, let p_F equal the number of unnecessary biopsies on the first screening divided by the number of subjects who received the first screening. Also let p_S equal the number of unnecessary biopsies on the second screening divided by the number of subjects who received the second screening. Over a period of 20 years the expected number of unnecessary biopsies is $u = p_F + 19 p_S$ with variance $\text{var}(u) = p_F(1 - p_F)/n + 19^2 p_S(1 - p_S)/n$, where n is the number of screened subjects.

4.10 Conclusion

PSE represents a novel approach to reducing selection bias when evaluating periodic cancer screening without a randomised control group. The main reduction in selection bias comes from estimating age-specific incidence in the absence of screening by using older screened subjects as controls for younger screened subjects. Simplified formulae for the variance and the sample size make the methodology easy to implement. However, before using PSE, one should think carefully about the assumptions to determine if they are reasonable.

References

Baker, S.G. (1989). Innovations in screening: Evaluating periodic screening without using data from a control group. In: *Advances in Cancer Control VI*, Engstrom, P.F., Anderson, P. and Mortenson, L. (eds), 15–21. Alan R. Liss, Inc., New York.

Baker, S.G. (1998). Evaluating the age to begin periodic breast cancer screening using data from a few regularly scheduled screens, *Biometrics*, **54**, 1569–78.

Baker, S.G. and Chu, K.C. (1990). Evaluating screening for the early detection and treatment of cancer without using a randomized control group. *Journal of the American Statistical Association*, **85**, 321–7.

Cox, D.R. and Oakes, D. (1984). *Analysis of Survival Data*, Chapman and Hall, London.

Elmore, J.G., Barton, M.B., Moceri, V.M., Polk, S., Arena, P.J. and Fletcher, S.W. (1998). Ten-year risk of false positive screening mammograms and clinical breast examinations. *The New England Journal of Medicine*, **338**, 1089–96.

Moran, M.K. (1998). Periodic screening evaluation under cohort effect. Master of Science Thesis, University of South Carolina.

Morrison, A.S., Brisson, J. and Khalid, N. (1988). Breast cancer incidence and mortality in the breast cancer detection demonstration project, *Journal of the National Cancer Institute*, **80**, 1540–7.

Prentice, R.L. (1989). Surrogate endpoints in clinical trials: definition and operating criteria. *Statistics in Medicine*, **8**, 431–40.

Shapiro, S., Venet, W., Strax, P. and Venet, L. (1988). *Periodic Screening for Breast Cancer. The Health Insurance Plan Project and Its Sequelae, 1963–1986*. Johns Hopkins University Press, Baltimore.

Appendix A: Derivation of age-specific incidence if no screening

Let F_0 denote a positive first screening at age a and detection in the interval if no first screening. Let F_1 denote a positive first screening at age a and detection on the second screen if no first screening. Therefore $q_F(a) = q_{F_0}(a) + q_{F_1}(a)$. In the absence of a first screening, the probability of detection in the interval is $q_N(A) = q_{F_0}(a) + q_I(a)$ and the probability of detection on the first screen at age $a + 1$ is $q_F(a + 1) = q_{F_1}(a) + q_S(a)$. Substituting $q_F(a)$, $q_N(a)$ and $q_F(a + 1)$ into (4.1) gives an identity. For a more formal proof see Baker (1998).

Appendix B: Variance approximation

Because the squares of the differences are sometimes relatively small, we approximate var(g) using only the last two terms from (4.5):

$$\mathrm{var}(g) = Q_I^2 (v_N + v_I) + Q_S^2 (v_N + v_S) \tag{B.1}$$

Because v_I is likely to be larger than v_S because it is based on fewer cases, we substitute v_I for v_S to conservatively approximate (B.1) as

$$\mathrm{var}(g) \approx (Q_I^2 + Q_S^2)(v_N + v_I) \tag{B.2}$$

Recall that $\alpha = Q_I/Q_N$. As an approximation we set $Q_S/Q_N = (1 - \alpha)$ and (B.2) reduces to

$$\mathrm{var}(g) \approx (\alpha^2 + (1 - \alpha)^2)Q_N^2 (v_N + v_I) \tag{B.3}$$

Recall that n is the number of screened subjects per age interval and π is the fraction who refuse screening. To compute v_I, we need the expected number per age interval of interval cancer cases, which is $Q_I n = \alpha Q_N n$. To compute v_M, we need the expected number of subjects who refuse screening, which is $Q_N n \pi (1 - \pi)$. These imply

$$v_N + v_I = \frac{m_N (1 - m_N)}{n Q_N \pi (1 - \pi)} + \frac{m_I (1 - m_I)}{n \alpha Q_N}$$

$$\leq \frac{1/4}{n Q_N \pi (1 - \pi)} + \frac{1/4}{n \alpha Q_N}$$

$$\leq \frac{1}{4 Q_N n} \left(\frac{1}{\alpha} + \frac{1 - \pi}{\pi} \right) \tag{B.4}$$

Substituting (B.4) into (B.3) gives (4.7).

Markov chain models of breast tumour progression and its arrest by screening

Stephen W. Duffy, Hsiu-Hsi Chen, Teresa C. Prevost and Laszlo Tabar

5.1 Tumour progression

In assessing the early detection of a disease through screening, a first model is often the following:

1. Every subject begins with no detectable disease at all. Some subjects will develop the disease of interest, some will remain free of the disease all their lives.
2. For a subject who develops disease, at a certain time t_0 the person will pass to a state where the disease is asymptomatic but can be detected by a screening test. This phase is often called the *preclinical detectable period* (PCDP).
3. For this subject, at a certain time t_1 ($t_1 > t_0$), the disease will become clinically symptomatic. In the absence of screening this is defined as the time of diagnosis (although in practice there may be a delay from symptoms to diagnosis). The period $t_1 - t_0$ is known as the *sojourn time*.

This basic model is described more fully and illustrated graphically in Chapter 1. In mammographic screening for breast cancer, the aim is to diagnose the disease at a stage when it is amenable to treatment. Tumours diagnosed earlier are more likely to be small, and less likely to have invaded the regional lymph nodes. Early detection has two potential benefits: first the greater likelihood of successful treatment and the avoidance of breast cancer death, and second the possibility of less aggressive or disfiguring treatment.

For screening in this context to be effective, the disease needs to be diagnosed some time before t_1, while it is treatable with less aggressive methods and while it is curable in the long term. This means that a substantial *lead time* and good *sensitivity* are required.

If we add a third time point to the above, t_2 ($t_1 > t_2 > t_0$), equal to the time of detection by screening, the lead time is defined as $t_1 - t_2$. Thus the lead time is the time by which screening advances the diagnosis from the time at which the tumour would have been diagnosed clinically. The sensitivity is the probability that a case of disease which is in the preclinical detectable phase is actually diagnosed by the screening test. The sensitivity (S) and the average length of the preclinical detectable period (*mean sojourn time*, MST) are therefore crucial parameters to the ability of screening to affect subsequent mortality from the disease.

A related concept which depends on sensitivity, mean sojourn time and the interval between screens is the *programme sensitivity*. This is the probability that a tumour arising in a population subjected to screening will be diagnosed at screening (as opposed to clinical occurrence in the interval between screens). Clearly, the better the performance of the screening programme, the higher the programme sensitivity. On the other hand, if the programme sensitivity is low, that is the proportion of tumours which arise in the interval between screens (*interval cancers*) is relatively high, this suggests that either the sojourn time is short or the screening test sensitivity poor.

5.2 Markov chain models

A commonly assumed distribution of time spent in a given state is the *exponential*. This has been shown to be useful in modelling the sojourn time in breast cancer. If the sojourn time is exponentially distributed, the form of the probability of a given tumour becoming clinical within a period t since its entry to the preclinical detectable period is $1 - e^{-\lambda t}$.

The parameter λ, to be estimated from the data, is the inverse of the mean of the distribution. Thus if λ^* is our estimate of λ, our estimate of mean sojourn time is $1/\lambda^*$. The seminal papers on this model of sojourn time are by Zelen and Feinleib (1969), Prorok (1976) and Day and Walter (1984).

An important property of the exponential distribution is that of 'no memory'. This is easiest to define in the context of the preclinical detectable period. It means that if the time spent in the preclinical detectable phase is exponentially distributed, and if it is known that a tumour is in that preclinical phase at time t, then the probability of transition to symptomatic clinical disease within a subsequent period is not dependent on the state of the tumour (no detectable disease or preclinical screen-detectable) at any time before time t. A corollary of this is that although the sojourn time is an upper limit on the lead time achievable, if sojourn time is assumed to be exponentially distributed, the expected lead time of a screen-diagnosed cancer is equal to the mean sojourn time.

The property that conditional on the state at a given time t, probabilities of subsequent events are independent of the event history before t is the fundamental and defining property of Markov chains. It is referred to as the Markov property hereafter. Formally, a Markov chain is a series of observed states in time, in which, conditional on the state at any time t, the probability of being in any state at time $t + h$ is independent of the states occupied prior to time t.

The model of no detectable disease, preclinical screen detectable disease and clinical disease, might be considered a three-state Markov chain. One might wish to expand this to a five-state Markov chain in which the preclinical and clinical phases were each divided into two states for node negative (not yet invaded the regional lymph nodes) and node positive (invaded the regional lymph nodes). In principle, there is no limit on the number of states, but the algebraic and computing complexity render it impractical to obtain estimates for numbers of states in excess of 10 without imposing substantial further assumptions.

The flexibility in terms of incorporation of states representing stage of disease progression (bearing in mind the practical limitations) is one of the advantages of the Markov chain model. Others include the ability to take account of aspects of disease progression and natural history in the evaluation of a screening programme, the estimation of parameters of the natural history from repeat observations on the same individuals (the Markov property is particularly useful here), and the ability to estimate transition probabilities even when the exact transition times are unobserved. The major drawback is that sometimes the Markov property cannot be assumed to hold, for instance if rapid progression in the past is a predictor of rapid progression in the future independent of the state of disease at present.

To demonstrate the use of the models and methods described below, we use data from the Swedish Two-County Trial of mammographic screening for breast cancer (Tabar *et al.*, 1995a). In this study, 77 080 women aged 40–74 were randomised to invitation to screening (Active Study Population, ASP), 55 985 to no invitation (Passive Study Population, PSP), for 7–8 years. Contemporaneously with the last screen of the ASP, the PSP had a single screen. Women aged 40–49 at randomisation were invited every 24 months, women aged 50 or more every 33 months, on average. Screening was abandoned after the second screen in women aged 70–74, due to poor attendance rates. The cancers diagnosed in the trial are shown by age and detection mode in Table 5.1. It should be borne in mind that pre-1995 publications of this study quote a slightly smaller number of cancers due to late registrations. Note the larger proportion of interval cancers in the age group 40–49, suggesting poorer sensitivity, shorter sojourn time (more rapid progression) or both, in this age group. This fundamental age difference will be further quantified by the methods described below. For the analyses demonstrated below we shall not use the 70–74 age group, since data are relatively sparse in this group.

Table 5.1 Cancers (%) diagnosed by age at randomisation and detection mode; Swedish Two-County Study

Detection mode	Age			
	40–49	50–59	60–69	70–74
ASP Prior*	6 (2)	5 (1)	13 (2)	4 (1)
ASP screen 1	39 (15)	103 (27)	184 (35)	101 (39)
ASP screen 2+	110 (43)	156 (41)	183 (35)	52 (20)
ASP interval	91 (36)	90 (24)	96 (18)	52 (20)
ASP refuser	10 (4)	28 (7)	53 (10)	50 (20)
Total ASP	**256**	**382**	**529**	**259**[†]
PSP pre-screen	115 (71)	221 (71)	277 (66)	142 (96)
PSP screen 1	47 (29)	94 (29)	140 (34)	6 (4)
Total PSP	**162**	**315**	**417**	**148**

* Prior = cancers diagnosed clinically between randomisation and first screen
[†] Includes 30 cancers diagnosed after screening was abandoned in this age group

5.3 Some simple estimates

It is possible to derive some simple estimates of mean sojourn time, sensitivity and programme sensitivity without formal mathematical modelling. First, define

P = the number of cases per thousand screened, diagnosed at the first (prevalence) screen;

I = the incidence of the disease per thousand persons per year in an unscreened population;

C_s = the number of cases detected by screening during a period of observation of a screening programme;

C_i = the number of clinical cases arising in the intervals between screening during the same period of observation; and

F_i = the total number of interval cases arising clinically within one year of a negative screen in the same period of observation.

Now, consider the mean sojourn time. If the mean sojourn time is x years, one would expect to anticipate approximately x years of disease incidence with a single screen of a population, assuming good sensitivity (Day *et al.*, 1989). Thus, assuming 100% sensitivity and no over-diagnosis, an estimate of the mean sojourn time is given by

$$MST = P/I$$

To obtain a simple estimate of sensitivity, further approximation is necessary. In the period after a population is screened, the cancers arising clinically in those screened negative will be of two types: cancers which were in the preclinical detectable period at the time of the screen but were missed at the screen; and cancers newly 'born' into the preclinical detectable period after the screen, and progressing to clinical disease before the next screen. It is not possible to distinguish these two groups with certainty, but it is reasonable to assume that the cancers arising clinically soon after the negative screen are mainly the missed cases, and those arising later are mainly truly new cancers. A possible estimate of test sensitivity is therefore:

$$S = \frac{C_s}{C_s + F_i}$$

This assumes that clinical cancers arising within one year of a negative screen constitute exclusively and exhaustively the population of cancers missed at the screen. This assumption is very unlikely to be true, but may be a reasonable approximation.

A simple estimate of the programme sensitivity is the observed proportion of cases which are screen-detected:

$$PS = \frac{C_s}{C_s + C_i}$$

A refinement to this might be to exclude the prevalence screen tumours and the interval cancers immediately following the prevalence screen from the formula for programme sensitivity; inclusion of the large number of prevalent cases may artificially inflate the sensitivity.

For an example of the estimates, we take the data from the ASP in the Swedish Two-County Trial in the age range 50–59. In this age group there were 103 cancers diagnosed at the first screen in 21 559 women attending for screening (see Table 5.2), giving P = 4.78 per thousand. The corresponding incidence in the unscreened control group was 1.87 per thousand per year (Tabar *et al.*, 1992). Thus the MST may be estimated as 4.78/1.87 = 2.55. From Table 5.1 there were 259 screen-detected cancers in all, and 90 interval cancers, giving a programme sensitivity of 259/349 = 74%. Eliminating the first screen and its associated interval cancers, we have an estimate of 156/218 = 72%. Of the interval cancers, 18 arose in the first year after a negative screen, giving as an estimate of screening test sensitivity 259/277 = 94%.

While these estimates are reasonable and useful, they involve approximations and assumptions which may not be true. For example the formula above for mean sojourn time assumes uniform incidence and progression, and 100% sensitivity. The more complex Markov modelling of the disease process may yield more realistic estimates.

5.4 Estimation from three-state Markov chain models

A simple example is a three-state model where states 0, 1 and 2 represent no detectable disease, preclinical screen-detectable disease and clinical symptomatic disease respectively. Associated with such a Markov model is a transition matrix of instantaneous probabilities of moving from state to state. Formally such a matrix is defined as follows: in row i and column j (i not equal to j) of the matrix will be the element λ_{ij} such that in an extremely

Table 5.2 Numbers screened, screen-detected and interval cancers for the first three rounds of screening in the age group 50–59, Swedish Two-County Study

Screening round	Category	Number of subjects[a]	Approximate PY for interval
1	Attended screen	21 559	
	Cancers at screen	103	
	Interval cancers 0–12 months	3	21 456[b]
	Interval cancers 13–24 months	12	21 453[c]
	Interval cancers 25+ months	13	16 081[d]
2	Attended screen	18 792	
	Cancers at screen	61	
	Interval cancers 0–12 months	7	18 731
	Interval cancers 13–24 months	11	18 724
	Interval cancers 25+ months	4	14 035
3	Attended screen	16 127	
	Cancers at screen	69	
	Interval cancers 0–12 months	8	16 058
	Interval cancers 13–24 months	14	16 050
	Interval cancers 25+ months	17	12 027

[a]One interval cancer with missing time to last screen excluded
[b]21 559 – 103 = 21 456
[c]21 456 – 3 = 21 453
[d](21 453 – 12) × 0.75 = 16 081

short period of time h, the probability of moving from state i to state j is $\lambda_{ij}h$. For $i = j$, the element λ_{ii} is such that the probability of staying in state i is $1 + \lambda_{ii}h$.

For the above three-state model we posit the following transition matrix:

$$
\begin{pmatrix}
-\lambda_1 & \lambda_1 & 0 \\
0 & -\lambda_2 & \lambda_2 \\
0 & 0 & 0
\end{pmatrix}
$$

λ_1 and λ_2 are known as the instantaneous rates of transition from no detectable disease to preclinical disease and from preclinical disease to clinical disease respectively. Thus λ_1 is the birth rate into the PCDP, and λ_2 is the transition rate from preclinical to clinical disease. We assume spontaneous regression to be impossible. We also assume that to reach the clinical phase, a tumour must pass through the preclinical. As mentioned above, a property of this model is that $1/\lambda_2$ is the MST. The instantaneous transition rates need to be converted into probabilities of transition in non-instantaneous periods of time, by solving a potentially complex set of algebraic equations known as the Kolmogorov equations. Standard matrix algebra methods are available to obtain the solution. The methodology is described by Cox and Miller (1965), and a demonstration is given by Kay (1986). In this simple model, the solution can be derived by hand, giving the formulae for probabilities of transition in a non-negligible time t as in the following *transition probability matrix*:

$$
\begin{pmatrix}
e^{-\lambda_1 t} & \dfrac{\lambda_1 (e^{-\lambda_2 t} - e^{-\lambda_1 t})}{(\lambda_1 - \lambda_2)} & 1 - \dfrac{(\lambda_1 e^{-\lambda_2 t} - \lambda_2 e^{-\lambda_1 t})}{(\lambda_1 - \lambda_2)} \\
0 & e^{-\lambda_2 t} & 1 - e^{-\lambda_2 t} \\
0 & 0 & 1
\end{pmatrix}
$$

The formula in row i and column j above is the probability of an individual's being in state j at time $T + t$ if that individual was in state i at time T. Note that the formulae depend on t, the time within which the transition takes place and not on T, the initial time.

The formulae may become further complicated when for example women with a previous history of clinical breast cancer are excluded from the programme (as is the case in the Two-County Trial), so we have to condition on this for probabilities pertaining to the first screen. Also, inclusion of false positive and false negative screening error probabilities render the probabilities very complex. In addition, data on incidence (second or subsequent) screens are frequently either unavailable or sparse. Prevost *et al.* (1998) derive some approximations to the probabilities which can be used to obtain estimates using only

1. numbers of interval cancers and person-years blocked into one-year periods since negative screen;
2. number of cancers detected and number screened at the prevalence screen; and
3. total number of screen-detected cancers at screens preceding the periods in which the interval cancers arose (frequently equal to the number of cancers in (2) above).

Table 5.2 shows the construction of this data from the ASP of the Two-County Trial, for the age group 50–59. Appendix A shows a SAS programme for non-linear least squares estimation of MST and S, using the approximations of Prevost *et al.* (1998). In this case, we obtain estimates of 0.33 (95% CI 0.24–0.41) for the rate of transition from preclinical to clinical disease, which translates into 3.03 years (95% CI 2.43–4.17) for the MST, and 100% (95% CI 89–100) for S. It is possible to incorporate incidence screen data, but it is interesting to see the method demonstrated without incidence screens, as often the user will wish to perform evaluation before incidence screen data are available.

It is also, of course, possible to use the exact times to diagnosis of interval cancers, the yield of cancers at individual incidence screens, and the exact likelihood as calculated from the transition probability matrix above. An example of this will be demonstrated in the next section.

5.5 Estimation from a five-state Markov chain model

Consider a model including axillary lymph node status. There are five states:

1. no detectable disease (0);
2. preclinical node negative (pre –);
3. preclinical node positive (pre +);
4. clinical node negative (clin –);
5. clinical node positive (clin +).

The transition matrix is:

$$\begin{pmatrix} -\lambda_1 & \lambda_1 & 0 & 0 & 0 \\ 0 & -\lambda_2 - \lambda_3 & \lambda_2 & \lambda_3 & 0 \\ 0 & 0 & -\lambda_4 & \lambda_4 & 0 \\ 0 & 0 & 0 & 0 & 0 \\ 0 & 0 & 0 & 0 & 0 \end{pmatrix}$$

We assume no regression as before, that all tumours are born node negative and in the preclinical phase, and that transition in two dimensions at exactly the same instant is not possible. Note that we cannot estimate transitions within the clinical phase, as once a tumour is diagnosed, it is excised and further assessment of natural history thereafter is impossible.

Increasing the number of states from three to five as in this case brings about increases in algebraic complexity. Hand solution of the Kolmogorov equations is somewhat rebarbative, so the following strategy may be implemented:

1. Use computer software for symbolic algebra, such as *Mathematica* (Wolfram, 1991), to solve the Kolmogorov equations to produce transition probabilities from the transition rates.
2. For each type of transition observed, calculate the expected number of transitions (symbolically), using (1) and the error probabilities, if these are also to be modelled.
3. Solve the equation

Observed transitions = expected transitions + error

as a non-linear regression.

Table 5.3 Results from fitting a five-state model for progression including node status to data from the age group 50–59, Swedish Two-County Study

Rate parameter	Estimate	95% confidence interval
0 pre −	0.00 177	0.00 173–0.00 180
pre − pre +	0.24	0.19–0.30
pre − clin −	0.18	0.12–0.23
pre + clin +	1.00	0.73–1.27

This means we do not actually maximise the likelihood but estimate the transition rates and error probabilities as a solution of a complex set of estimating equations. With suitable weighting, these give approximations to maximum likelihood estimates assuming that counts of events are distributed as Poisson random variables. For further details of algebra and statistical methods see Chen *et al.* (1996, 1997a). Appendix B shows a SAS programme and data format for carrying out such analysis. Note the increased coding burden associated with the expansion of the number of states.

Table 5.3 shows the estimated instantaneous transition rates, again using the age group 50–59 in the Swedish Two-County Study. From these, absolute probabilities of progression within non-instantaneous intervals can be calculated. For example, a tumour which is preclinical and node negative at any point in time has a 22% chance of becoming clinical (either node negative or node positive), a 19% chance of becoming node positive (preclinical or clinical) and an 8% chance of becoming clinical and node positive within one year. For a tumour which is preclinical and node positive, the probability of becoming clinical within a year is 63%.

5.6 Application to age differences in progression and design of screening programmes

Table 5.4 shows the estimated incidence, mean sojourn time and sensitivity and positive predictive value from a three-state (no detectable disease, preclinical disease, clinical disease) model. The clear implications are that sensitivity is poorer and that progression of the disease to the clinical phase is faster in women aged under 50. As stated above, the programme sensitivity (the proportion of tumours which will be picked up by screening) depends on the screening sensitivity, the sojourn time and the interval between screens.

Table 5.4 Estimated incidence per 100 000 person-years, mean sojourn time (MST) and sensitivity by age, Swedish Two-County Study

	Estimate (95% CI) for age group		
Parameter	40–49	50–59	60–69
Preclinical incidence	89 (84–95)	155 (150–160)	240 (230–251)
MST in years	2.44 (2.12–2.86)	3.70 (3.44–4.17)	4.17 (4.00–4.55)
Sensitivity as %	83 (76–91)	100 (–)	100 (–)

The form of the dependence, given by Launoy *et al.* (1998) under the three-state Markov model, with S being the sensitivity, r the interval between screens and λ_2 the rate of progression from preclinical to clinical disease, is

$$PS = \frac{S(1 - e^{-\lambda_2 r})}{\lambda_2 r(1 - (1 - S)e^{-\lambda_2 r})}$$

Using this formula, the estimates of programme sensitivity by age and interscreening interval are shown in Table 5.5. These results indicate that around 80% programme sensitivity can be achieved by two-yearly screening in the age group 50–69, but only by annual screening in women aged under 50 years.

Table 5.6 shows estimated annual probabilities of progression with respect to node status and preclinical/clinical status by age, by applying the five-state model in 5.4 to age groups 40–49, 50–59 and 60–69. Again, the broad implications are that progression is considerably faster in the youngest age group. In particular, the very high probability of transition to clinical phase from node positive disease in the 40–49 age group shows that there is very little remaining scope for screening to advance the time of diagnosis in this age group once the tumour has invaded the regional lymph nodes. Similar results are obtained for a model based on tumour size or malignancy grade (a measure of a tumour's aggressive potential based on certain microscopic features), and for higher order models incorporating several factors simultaneously.

The above results all indicate a more rapid progression of tumours with respect to preclinical/clinical status, size and node status in the 40–49 age group. These factors are strongly associated with survival, in that poorer survival is associated with larger tumours, positive lymph node status and poorer malignancy grade. It is of some value to quantify this further, in terms of the mortality expected from different screening frequencies. We

Table 5.5 Estimated programme sensitivity by age group for different interscreening intervals

| Age group | Programme sensitivity (as percentage) with interscreening interval | | | |
	1 year	2 years	3 years	4 years
40–49	77	61	50	42
50–59	88	78	69	61
60–69	89	80	72	65

Table 5.6 Some estimated probabilities of progression with respect to preclinical/clinical status and node status, by age group

| Age | Probability of progression from/to clinical node + within one year, from state | |
	Preclinical node –	Preclinical node +
40–49	0.16	0.88
50–59	0.07	0.63
60–69	0.05	0.54

Table 5.7 Predicted percentage reduction in mortality from breast cancer by age group and interscreening interval (observed reduction in the Two-County Study given in parentheses)

Interscreening interval	Percentage mortality reduction in age group		
	40–49	50–59	60–69
1 year	36	46	44
2 years	18 (13)	39	39
3 years	4	34 (34)	34 (40)

use the data from the 2468 tumours in the Two-County Study to predict mortality as follows:

1. Using the Markov models, we estimate the numbers of tumours by node status, size and malignancy grade in an unscreened population and in a population screened every x years.
2. Use survival data from the 2468 tumours to estimate the 10-year (say) survival probability in each combination of the three factors.
3. Multiply the expected numbers of tumours in each category by the proportion expected to die of breast cancer in that category, to give the expected 10-year mortality.
4. Obtain predicted relative mortality by dividing the predicted mortality for the screened population by that for the unscreened.

Table 5.7 shows the predicted reduction in mortality using a model incorporating both size and node status. The effects of annual, two-yearly and three-yearly screening are given. It is assumed that 90% of those invited attend for screening (the approximate attendance rate observed in the Two-County Study), and the sensitivities estimated in Table 5.4 are used. Major points to note are that the predicted effects are close to those observed in the Two-County Study, that again, a shorter interscreening interval is required in the age group 40–49, and that the interval is less crucial for older women.

5.7 Some implications

The above demonstrates that it is feasible to combine screening data and Markov models to obtain estimates of disease progression using standard software, in this case SAS. The approach has been demonstrated using breast cancer screening in the examples above, but it is in principle applicable to screening for other diseases. From a statistical point of view, it is interesting to be able to estimate transition rates even though the times of transitions are not observed. If we detect a cancer at a screen, it is known to be in the preclinical phase at that screen, but we cannot tell at what exact time since the previous screen it actually entered the preclinical phase.

The results may have value in enhancing our understanding of the natural history of the disease, and they have clear implications for design of screening programmes. For example, they show that an interscreening interval of 2–3 years is sufficient to achieve a substantial mortality reduction in women aged 50 or more, but that an interval of at most 2 years, and preferably shorter, is required in women aged 40–49.

The approach above also has implications for study design. Firstly, the Markov models and predicted mortality methods may be used for power and sample size calculations. Secondly, because of the greater information, predicted mortality from tumours diagnosed has a lower variance than observed mortality. We might therefore consider using the predicted mortality from the tumours diagnosed as a surrogate in studies to evaluate different breast cancer screening strategies, although actual mortality would be necessary to establish the principle of screening in the first place. Predicted mortality is to be used in the case of the UK Breast Screening Frequency Trial, and has resulted in a study with a power double that which it would have had if based on actual mortality (Day and Duffy, 1996). The other advantage of use of predicted mortality is that it provides a result of the study some 10 years in advance of the observed mortality. This is particularly relevant to the case of breast cancer screening in the age group 40–49, where the actual mortality effect is distant in time, but the need for an answer is relatively urgent.

5.8 Other applications and further reading

Markov chain models can be applied to other diseases, including colorectal cancer (see Chapter 13), cervical cancer (Chapter 11), nasopharyngeal cancer (Chen et al., 1999), coronary heart disease (Sharples, 1993), AIDS (Satten and Longini, 1996) and cataract progression in diabetes (Prevost et al., 1999). Similar but non-Markov models have been applied to screening for retinoblastoma in infants (see Chapter 14). The methods have been extended to incorporate covariates (Prevost et al., 1999; Marshall and Jones, 1995), to evaluation using case-control designs (Chapter 11), and for estimation in the absence of interval cancer data (Lai et al., 1998).

The estimation algorithm used here is by no means the only one available. Originally, Chen et al. (1997a) proposed an unweighted non-linear least squares solution, but after criticism of the fit of the estimates, refined this to the weighted version described above (van den Akker-van Marle et al., 1998; Chen et al., 1998). Other possibilities include generalised linear models (Paci and Duffy, 1991), maximum likelihood (Day and Walter, 1984), microsimulation techniques (de Koning et al., 1995) and Markov chain Monte Carlo, a Bayesian stochastic estimation technique which is very powerful for estimation from complex models (Sharples, 1993; Satten and Longini, 1996; Prevost et al., 1999). For the mathematical background on stochastic processes, including Markov chain models, the classic text is by Cox and Miller (1965).

The methods have been extended beyond the evaluation of screening programmes. Applications include the design of studies (Chen et al., 1999), assessment of disease progression rates for purposes of better understanding of natural history (Satten and Longini, 1996; Sharples, 1993), and the effects of covariates on these progression rates (Marshall and Jones, 1995; Prevost et al. 1999). A specialist application is the use of these models to assess the issue of phenotypic drift or dedifferentiation in breast cancer. There is evidence that at least in some breast tumours, the malignancy grade deteriorates as a tumour develops. Chen et al. (1997b) applied a model in which an unknown proportion of tumours may progress with respect to malignancy grade states, and the remaining tumours may not, and estimated the unknown proportion of 'movers' for different age groups.

In terms of breast cancer progression and its arrest by screening, the assessment of the likely impact on mortality of different screening intervals is discussed more fully by Chen *et al.* (1997c). The validation in independent studies of the prediction of mortality from the size, node status and malignancy grade of the tumours diagnosed is given in the report on the historic Falun meeting on mammographic screening in women aged 40–49 (Organizing Committee and Collaborators, 1996). Corroborative evidence of the more rapid progression in younger women in the form of the histologic types of disease diagnosed in different age groups is given by Tabar *et al.* (1995b). Fuller details of the phenotypic drift issue are given by Tabar *et al.* (1996).

References

Chen, H.H., Duffy, S.W. and Tabar, L. (1996). A Markov chain method to estimate the tumour progression rate from preclinical to clinical phase, sensitivity and positive predictive value for mammography in breast cancer screening. *The Statistician*, **45**, 307–17.

Chen, H.H., Duffy, S.W., Tabar, L. and Day, N.E. (1997a). Markov chain models for progression of breast cancer, Part I: Tumour attributes and the preclinical detectable phase. *Journal of Epidemiology and Biostatistics*, **2**, 9–23.

Chen, H.H., Duffy, S.W. and Tabar, L. (1997b). A mover–stayer mixture of Markov chain models for the assessment of dedifferentiation and tumour progression in breast cancer. *Journal of Applied Statistics*, **24**, 265–78.

Chen, H.H., Duffy, S.W., Tabar, L. and Day, N.E. (1997c). Markov chain models for progression of breast cancer, Part II: Prediction of outcomes for different screening regimes. *Journal of Epidemiology and Biostatistics*, **2**, 25–35.

Chen, H.H., Duffy, S.W., Tabar, L. and Day, N.E. (1998). Reply. *Journal of Epidemiology and Biostatistics*, **3**, 424–7.

Chen, H.H., Prevost, T.C. and Duffy, S.W. (1999). Evaluation of screening for nasopharyngeal carcinoma: trial design using Markov chain models. *British Journal of Cancer*, **79**, 1894–1900.

Cox, D.R. and Miller, H.D. (1965). *The Theory of Stochastic Processes*. Methuen, London.

Day, N.E. and Walter, S.D. (1984). Simplified models of screening for chronic disease: estimation procedures from mass screening programmes. *Biometrics*, **43**, 1–13.

Day, N.E. and Duffy, S.W. (1996). Trial design based on surrogate end points – application to comparison of different breast screening frequencies. *Journal of the Royal Statistical Society A*, **159**, 49–60.

Day, N.E., Williams, D.R.R. and Khaw, K.T. (1989). Breast cancer screening programmes: the development of a monitoring and evaluation system. *British Journal of Cancer*, **59**, 954–8.

de Koning, H.J., Boer, R., Warmerdam, P.G., Beemsterboer, P.M.M. and van der Maas, P.J. (1995). Quantitative interpretation of age-specific mortality reductions from the Swedish breast cancer screening trials. *Journal of the National Cancer Institute*, **87**, 1217–23.

Kay, R. (1986). A Markov model for analysing cancer markers and disease states in survival studies. *Biometrics*, **42**, 855–65.

Lai, M.S., Yen, M.F., Kuo, H.S., Koong, S.L., Chen, T.H.H. and Duffy, S.W. (1998). Efficacy of breast-cancer screening for female relatives of breast-cancer-index cases: Taiwan Multicentre Cancer Screening (TAMCAS). *International Journal of Cancer*, **78**, 21–6.

Launoy, G., Duffy, S.W., Prevost, T.C. and Bouvier, V. (1998). Depistage des cancers: sensibilite du test et de la procedure de depistage. *Revue d'Epidemiologie et de Sante Publique*, **46**, 420–6.

Marshall, G. and Jones, R.H. (1995). Multi-state models and diabetic retinopathy. *Statistics in Medicine*, **14**, 1975–83.

Organizing Committee and Collaborators, Falun Meeting (1996). Breast cancer screening with mammography in women aged 40–49 years. *International Journal of Cancer*, **68**, 693–9.

Paci, E. and Duffy, S.W. (1991). Modelling the analysis of breast cancer screening programmes: sensitivity, lead time and predictive value in the Florence District Programme (1975–1986). *International Journal of Epidemiology*, **20**, 852–8.

Prevost, T.C., Launoy, G., Duffy, S.W. and Chen, H.H. (1998). Estimating sensitivity and sojourn time in screening for colorectal cancer: a comparison of statistical approaches. *American Journal of Epidemiology*, **148**, 609–19.

Prevost, T.C., Rohan, T.E., Duffy, S.W., Chen, H.H., To, T. and Hill, R.D. (1999). Markov chain models and estimation of absolute progression rates: application to cataract progression in diabetic adults. *Journal of Epidemiology and Biostatistics*, **4**, 337–44.

Prorok, P.C. (1976). The theory of periodic screening II. Doubly bounded recurrence times and mean time and detection probability estimation. *Advances in Applied Probability*, **8**, 460–76.

Satten, G.A. and Longini, I.M. (1996). Markov chains with measurement error: estimating the 'true' course of the human immunodeficiency virus disease. *Applied Statistics*, **45**, 275–95.

Sharples, L.D. (1993). Use of the Gibbs sampler to estimate transition rates between grades of coronary disease following cardiac transplantation. *Statistics in Medicine*, **12**, 1155–69.

Tabar, L., Fagerberg, G., Duffy, S.W., Day, N.E., Gad, A. and Grontoft, O. (1992). Update of the Swedish Two-County program of mammographic screening for breast cancer. *Radiologic Clinics of North America*, **30**, 187–210.

Tabar, L., Fagerberg, G., Chen, H.H., Duffy, S.W., Smart, C.R., Gad, A. and Smith, R.A. (1995a). Efficacy of breast cancer screening by age: new results from the Swedish Two-County trial. *Cancer*, **75**, 2507–17.

Tabar, L., Fagerberg, G., Chen, H.H., Duffy, S.W. and Gad, A. (1995b). Screening for breast cancer in women aged under 50: mode of detection, incidence and histology. *Journal of Medical Screening*, **2**, 94–8.

Tabar, L., Fagerberg, G., Chen, H.H., Duffy, S.W. and Gad, A. (1996). Tumour development, histology and grade of breast cancers: prognosis and progression. *International Journal of Cancer*, **66**, 413–19.

van den Akker-van Marle, M.E., Boer, R. and van Oortmarssen, G.J. (1998). Comments on Duffy/Chen Markov chain models for progression of breast cancer. *Journal of Epidemiology and Biostatistics*, **3**, 423–4.

Wolfram, S. (1991). *Mathematica: A System for Doing Mathematics by Computer*. Addison-Wesley, Redwood City, California.

Zelen, M. and Feinleib, M. (1969). On the theory of screening for chronic disease. *Biometrika*, **56**, 601–14.

Appendix A: Software for estimation of MST and *S* from a three-state model

```
/*
THIS SAS PROGRAM TAKES INTERVAL CANCER DATA AND PREVALENCE
SCREEN-DETECTED CANCER DATA AS BELOW AND ESTIMATES LAM, THE
RATE OF PROGRESSION FROM PRECLINICAL TO CLINICAL DISEASE (AND
HENCE THE RECIPROCAL OF THE MEAN SOJOURN TIME), AND SCREENING
SENSITIVITY. THE DATA ARE READ IN AS TIME SINCE LAST SCREEN
(AVERAGE AGE FOR PREVALENCE SCREEN), INDICATOR OF SCREEN
DETECTION (0=INTERVAL, 1=PREVALENCE SCREEN), INDICATOR OF
INTERVAL CANCER (0=SCREEN DETECTED, 1=INTERVAL), NUMBER OF
CANCERS, PERSON-YEARS (OR NUMBER SCREENED IF THESE ARE SCREEN
DETECTED CANCERS). THE DATA ARE BLOCKED INTO WHOLE YEARS. IN
THE EXAMPLE BELOW, THE TIME VARIABLE IS GIVEN AS 0.5 FOR THE
FIRST YEAR, 1.5 FOR THE SECOND AND 2.375 FOR THE THIRD (IN
THIS SCREENING PROGRAMME, THE AVERAGE SCREENING INTERVAL WAS
2.75 YEARS).
THE ESTIMATION PROCEDURE IS A QUASI-LIKELIHOOD NON-LINEAR LEAST
SQUARES. THE WEIGHTING MEANS THAT THE ANSWER IS AN
APPROXIMATION TO A MLE WHERE THE EVENTS ARE A POISSON PROCESS
*/
data m;
   input time scr int obs py;
cards;
0.5 0 1 3 21456
1.5 0 1 12 21453
2.375 0 1 13 16081
0.5 0 1 7 18731
1.5 0 1 11 18724
2.375 0 1 4 14035
0.5 0 1 8 16058
1.5 0 1 14 16050
2.375 0 1 17 12027
55 1 0 103 21559
  ;
run;

data s;
   set m;
/*
NB THE PROGRAM ALSO REQUIRES YOU TO PUT IN THE UNDERLYING
INCIDENCE OF THE DISEASE AND THE TOTAL NUMBER OF
SCREEN-DETECTED CANCERS BELOW
*/
inc=0.00187;
can=233;

run;
```

```
proc nlin method=dud data=s maxiter=200 g4singular;

parms lam=0.3
      sen=0.9
      ;

bounds 0 < sen <= 1;
bounds 0.1 < lam < 5;

e=inc*py;
p00=(inc*(exp(-inc*time)-exp(-lam*time))/(lam-inc))*sen
/(exp(-inc*time)+(inc*(exp(-inc*time)-exp(-lam*time))/
  (lam-inc)));

if _iter_=-1 then do;
_weight_=1;
end;
else do;
_weight_=1/sqrt((int*(e*(1-exp(-lam*time))))+(can*((1-sen)/sen)*
(exp(-lam*(time-0.5))-exp(-lam*(time+0.5))))))+(scr*py*p00));
end;

model obs=(int*(e*(1-exp(-lam*time))))+(can*((1-sen)/sen)*
(exp(-lam*(time-0.5))-exp(-lam*(time+0.5))))))+(scr*py*p00);

resid=obs-model.obs;
output out=c r=resid p=fitted;

run;

data c;
set c;
e=inc*py;
proc print;
run;
```

Appendix B: SAS program to estimate transition rates from a five-state model for node status

```
data node50;

/*
  This program estimates
  b1:Hazard rate for transition from no to pre_N(-)
  b2:Hazard rate for transition from pre_N(-) to pre_N(+)
  b3:Hazard rate for transition from pre_N(-) to clin_N(-)
  b4:Hazard rate for transition from pre_N(+) to clin_N(+)

    */

  infile '/home5/stephen/tony/node50a.dat';
```

```
   input how time no_first no_later
      first_1 first_2 later_1 later_2 clin_1 clin_2
      m_first mfirst_1 mfirst_2 mclin_1 mclin_2
      number agegp nodes m;
/* Data are read in free format as:
detection mode (not used)
time in months since last screen (age if this is first screen)
Then indicator variables for:
   first screen no cancer (0 if no, 1 if yes)
   later screen no cancer (ditto)
   first screen node negative cancer (ditto)
   first screen node positive cancer (ditto)
   later screen node negative cancer (ditto)
   later screen node positive cancer (ditto)
   interval cancer node negative cancer (ditto)
   interval cancer node positive cancer (ditto)
   control group first screen no cancer (ditto- if no control
      group, always 0)
   control group first screen node neg (ditto- if no control
      group, always 0)
   control group first screen node pos (ditto- if no control
      group, always 0)
   control group clinical node neg (ditto- if no control group,
      always 0)
   control group clinical node pos (ditto- if no control group,
      always 0)
   number of subjects in category
   age group (not used)
   node status (not used)
   age at first screen of control group, if control, 0 otherwise
      (if no control group, always 0).

Data look like

11 660 1 0 0 0 0 0 0 0 0 0 0 0 0 0 21457 1 9 0
11 33 0 1 0 0 0 0 0 0 0 0 0 0 0 0 34789 1 9 0
12 96 0 0 0 0 0 0 0 0 1 0 0 0 0 14385 1 9 660
1 660 0 0 1 0 0 0 0 0 0 0 0 0 0 80 1 0 0
1 660 0 0 0 1 0 0 0 0 0 0 0 0 0 19 1 1 0
2 33 0 0 0 0 1 0 0 0 0 0 0 0 0 105 1 0 0
2 33 0 0 0 0 0 1 0 0 0 0 0 0 0 21 1 1 0
3 3 0 0 0 0 0 0 1 0 0 0 0 0 0 1 1 0 0
3 5 0 0 0 0 0 0 1 0 0 0 0 0 0 2 1 0 0
3 6 0 0 0 0 0 0 1 0 0 0 0 0 0 3 1 0 0
3 7 0 0 0 0 0 0 1 0 0 0 0 0 0 1 1 0 0
3 8 0 0 0 0 0 0 1 0 0 0 0 0 0 1 1 0 0
3 12 0 0 0 0 0 0 1 0 0 0 0 0 0 1 1 0 0

and so on

*/
```

```
   proc print;

   run;

   data m;

   set node50;

   time=time/12;
   m=m/12;

run;

proc nlin method=dud data=m maxiter=200 g4singular;

parms  b1=0.0014
       b2=0.234
       b3=0.10
       b4=1.034


           ;
bounds 0 < b1 < 5;
bounds 0 < b2 < 5;
bounds 0 < b3 < 5;
bounds 0 < b4 < 5;

   if (b1 ne 0) and (b2 ne 0) and (b3 ne 0) and (b4 ne 0)


     ;

t1=time-0.08;

t2=0.08;

array  t{4}  time t1 t2 m;
array  v00{4}    p00 p_00 p00_ p00m;
array  v01{4}    p01 p_01 p01_ p01m;
array  v02{4}    p02 p_02 p02_ p02m;
array  v03{4}    p03 p_03 p03_ p03m;
array  v04{4}    p04 p_04 p04_ p04m;
array  v11{4}    p11 p_11 p11_ p11m;
array  v12{4}    p12 p_12 p12_ p12m;
array  v13{4}    p13 p_13 p13_ p13m;
array  v14{4}    p14 p_14 p14_ p14m;
array  v22{4}    p22 p_22 p22_ p22m;
array  v24{4}    p24 p_24 p24_ p24m;

do i=1 to 4;

v00{i}=Exp(-(b1*t{i}));
v01{i}=-(b1/((b1-b2-b3)*Exp(b1*t{i})))+
   b1/((b1-b2-b3)*Exp((b2+b3)*t{i}));
```

```
v02{i}=((b1*b2)/((b1-b2-b3)*(b2+b3-b4))-
       (b1*b2)/((b1-b4)*(b2+b3-b4)))/Exp(b1*t{i})
   -(b1-b2)/
  ((b1-b2-b3)*(b2+b3-b4)*
    Exp((b2+b3)*t{i}))+
  (b1*b2)/((b1-b4)*(b2+b3-b4)*Exp(b4*t{i})));
v03{i}=b3/(b2+b3)+(-(b3/(b2+b3))+
    (b1*b3)/((b1-b2-b3)*(b2+b3)))/Exp(b1*t{i})
  -(b1*b3)/
  ((b1-b2-b3)*(b2+b3)*Exp((b2+b3)*t{i}));
v04{i}=b2/(b2+b3)+(-(b2/(b2+b3))+
       (b1*b2)/((b1-b2-b3)*(b2+b3))-
       (b1*b2)/((b1-b2-b3)*(b2+b3-b4))+
       (b1*b2)/((b1-b4)*(b2+b3-b4)))/Exp(b1*t{i})
    +(b1*(-(b2/(b2+b3))+b2/(b2+b3-b4)))/
    ((b1-b2-b3)*Exp((b2+b3)*t{i}))-
  ((b1*b2)/((b1-b4)*(b2+b3-b4)*Exp(b4*t{i})));
v11{i}=Exp(-((b2+b3)*t{i}));
v12{i}=-(b2/((b2+b3-b4)*Exp((b2+b3)*t{i})))+
  b2/((b2+b3-b4)*Exp(b4*t{i})));
v13{i}=b3/(b2+b3)-b3/((b2+b3)*Exp((b2+b3)*t{i}));
v14{i}=b2/(b2+b3)+(-(b2/(b2+b3))+
    b2/(b2+b3-b4))*Exp((b2+b3)*t(i))-
  b2/((b2+b3-b4)*Exp(b4*t{i}));
v22{i}=Exp(-(b4*t{i}));
v24{i}=1-Exp(-(b4*t{i}));

end;

pc1=p00/(p00+p01+p02);

pc2=p00;

pc3=p01/(p00+p01+p02);

pc4=p01;

pc5=p02/(p00+p01+p02);

pc6=p02;


pc7=p_00*p03_+p_01*p13_;

pc8=p_00*p04_ +p_01*p14_+p_02*p24_;

pcm1=p00m*p00/(p00m+p01m+p02m);

pcm2=(p00m*p01+p01m*p11)/(p00m+p01m+p02m);

pcm3=(p00m*p02+p01m*p12+p02m*p22)/(p00m+p01m+p02m);
```

```
pcm4=(p00m*p_00*p03_+p00m*p_01*p13_+p01m*p_11*p13_)/(p00m+
      p01m+p02m);

pcm5=(p00m*p_00*p04_+p00m*p_01*p14_+p00m*p_02*p24_+
      p01m*p_11*p14_+ p01m*p_12*p24_
      +p02m*p_22*p24_)/(p00m+p01m+p02m);
if _iter_=-1 then do;
_weight_=1/sqrt(number);
end;
else do;
_weight_=1/sqrt(21559*no_first*pc1-21559*first_1*pc3+21559*
            first_2*pc5+34919*no_later*pc2-34919*later_1*pc4+34919*later_2*pc6
            +56246*clin_1*pc7+56246*clin_2*pc8+14699*pcm1*m_first+
            14699*pcm2*mfirst_1+14699*pcm3*mfirst_2+14699*
            pcm4*mclin_1+14699*pcm5*mclin_2);
end;
  model number=21559*no_first*pc1-21559*first_1*pc3+21559*first_2*pc5
            +34919*no_later*pc2-34919*later_1*pc4+34919*later_2*pc6
            +56246*clin_1*pc7+56246*clin_2*pc8+14699*pcm1*m_first
            -14699*pcm2*mfirst_1+14699*pcm3*mfirst_2+14699*pcm4*mclin_1
            -14699*pcm5*mclin_2;

resid=number-model.number;

output out=c r=resid p=fitted

run;

data c;

   set c;

proc print;

run;
```

6

Metastases at diagnosis: a key to understanding the natural history of breast cancer

Serge Koscielny, Ariane Auquier and Catherine Hill

6.1 Introduction

Among the subgroups of breast cancers defined on the basis of tumour volume, ranging from non-palpable lesions detected early by mammography to very bulky masses, some will be cured simply by local treatment. The proportion of patients cured merely with local treatment varies according to the tumour size. This variation could be interpreted as a result of the existence of a size beyond which each tumour will give birth to cells able to metastasise. The distribution of tumour volumes at the initiation of metastasis has been characterised by Koscielny *et al.* (1984). In breast cancer, the initiation of the first metastasis is a critical event in tumour progression.

A second important event occurs when metastases become detectable. However, most of the tumours are diagnosed and treated before this second event. Moreover, patients with detectable metastases at the time of diagnosis are systematically excluded from studies investigating prognostic factors. For the clinician, these patients are special cases, requiring systemic therapy and for whom the die is cast.

The existence of a relationship at the population level between the proportion of patients with distant metastases and the subsequent overall breast cancer mortality might seem obvious for the clinician. However the nature of this relationship has not been adequately investigated.

We hypothesise that the only difference between patients with detectable metastases at diagnosis and patients with occult metastases is the size of the metastases, which in the latter group are simply not large enough to be clinically detectable. On the basis of this postulate, we demonstrate theoretical relationships between the probability of metastases at diagnosis and in the long term. The clinical relevance of such relationships is examined and the implications for the natural history of breast cancer are discussed.

6.2 Patients and methods

6.2.1 Population studied

The population of patients studied included practically all cases of invasive breast carcinoma treated at the Institute Gustave-Roussy (IGR) from 1 January 1954 to 31 December 1975. The only exclusion criteria were male sex, previous treatment and bilateral primary tumours. A total of 4144 patients were included in this study. The treatment protocol did not change markedly during the entire period and has previously been described (Lacour *et al.*, 1968). In particular, adjuvant chemotherapy was not used.

The follow-up has been updated regularly and has potentially attained at least 20 years for all the patients. The dates of the first distant metastasis, first local relapse (LR), second malignancy (SM), controlateral breast cancer (CBC) and death were recorded. Only 204 patients were lost to follow-up within the first 20 years after treatment of the primary tumour.

6.2.2 Characteristics studied

The clinical tumour diameter was available for 3915 patients (94% of the population) with clinically unifocal tumours. The clinical tumour volume was estimated from the diameter, assuming that the tumour is a sphere. Eight categories of patients were defined as a function of the clinical tumour diameter, from less than 3 cm to 9 cm or more, with 1 cm increments between diameters (Table 6.1). These categories were known before initial treatment, independently of knowledge of the metastasis status. It should be noted that these tumours date from the premammography epoch and hence contain substantial numbers of large cancers.

6.2.3 Estimation of the proportions of patients with metastases

The proportion of patients by size category with detectable metastases at the time of diagnosis is given in Table 6.1. The cumulative probability of metastasis 20 years after diagnosis was estimated by the actuarial method without excluding patients with metastases at diagnosis (Figure 6.1). Events other than distant metastases (i.e. local recurrences, second malignancies or controlateral breast cancers) were ignored and patients who died free of distant metastases were censored at the date of death.

6.2.4 Quantitative methods

The mathematical aspects of the paper are developed in the appendix and can be summarised as follows. We assume exponential growth of both the primary tumour and the distant metastases, and proportionality between the doubling times. In a log–probit co-ordinate system (Finney, 1964), the relationship between the tumour volume at diagnosis (V_d) and

Table 6.1 Proportion of patients with metastasis at diagnosis of breast cancer and after 20 years of follow-up according to tumour volume at diagnosis. When the variability of V_d is ignored (last column), the predicted proportions in the long term are computed by adding 1.62 to the probit of the proportion of patients with metastases at diagnosis. The fit is satisfactory in groups of patients defined according to tumour volume, but not in the total population. A satisfactory fit is obtained in all the groups when the variability of V_d is taken into account. For the total population, this corresponds to the addition of 1.38 to the probit of the proportion of patients with metastases at diagnosis

Diameter D in cm	Tumour volume $V = \pi D^3/6$ in ml	Number of patients (% of total)	Proportion of patients with metastases			
			Estimation from the data		Prediction (*) in the long term,	
			At diagnosis (95% CI)	After 20 years of follow-up (95% CI)	Taking into account the variability of V_d	Ignoring the variability of V_d
<3	<14.1	591 (14%)	0.02 (0.01–0.03)	0.32 (0.28–0.36)	***0.31***	***0.35***
3–3.9	14.1– 33.4	779 (19%)	0.03 (0.02–0.05)	0.43 (0.39–0.47)	***0.42***	***0.42***
4–4.9	33.5– 65.3	747 (18%)	0.06 (0.04–0.08)	0.53 (0.49–0.57)	***0.52***	***0.52***
5–5.9	65.4–113.0	577 (14%)	0.09 (0.06–0.11)	0.59 (0.54–0.63)	***0.60***	***0.60***
6–6.9	113.1–179.5	427 (10%)	0.14 (0.11–0.17)	0.70 (0.65–0.74)	***0.70***	***0.71***
7–7.9	179.6–268.0	259 (6%)	0.22 (0.17–0.27)	0.79 (0.74–0.85)	***0.80***	***0.80***
8–8.9	268.1–381.6	169 (4%)	0.25 (0.18–0.31)	0.83 (0.76–0.89)	***0.83***	***0.83***
9+	≥ 381.7	366 (9%)	0.42 (0.37–0.47)	0.94 (0.91–0.97)	***0.92***	***0.92***
Missing or plurifocal	–	229 (6%)	0.07 (0.04–0.11)	0.48 (0.41–0.55)	not estimable	0.57
Total	–	4 144 (100%)	0.11 (0.10–0.12)	0.56 (0.55–0.58)	***0.56*** (†)	0.66

(*) Figures in bold italics correspond to predictions within the 95% confidence interval of the estimations

(†) Variability of V_d calculated using the 3915 patients with known tumour size

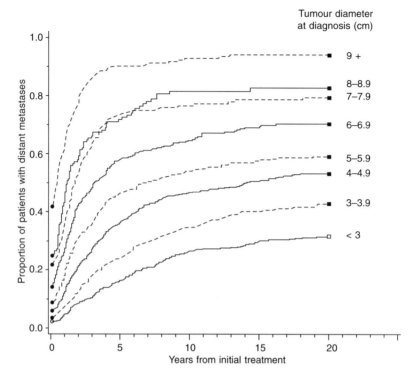

Figure 6.1 Cumulative proportion of patients with distant metastases as a function of time from initial treatment (actuarial method), in eight groups of patients defined according to tumour diameter at diagnosis. Patients with detectable metastases at diagnosis are included

the proportion of patients with metastases at diagnosis is expected to be parallel to the relationship between V_d and the cumulated proportion of patients with metastases 20 years after treatment. This parallelism results from the constancy of the number of tumour volume doublings between the tumour volume at metastasis initiation (V_0) and at metastasis detection (V_1). As a consequence of this parallelism the probability of metastases at long term can be extrapolated from the proportion of patients with detectable distant metastases at diagnosis.

Assuming Gompertzian growth (Gratton *et al.*, 1978) for the tumour and the metastases, the two curves are expected to rejoin at a point corresponding to the maximum asymptotic tumour volume (tumour volume which would be reached after an infinite duration of growth).

6.3 Results

6.3.1 Relationship between the tumour volume and the probability of metastases

The relationships between the tumour volume and the proportion of patients with metastases at diagnosis and with metastases after 20 years of follow-up are plotted in Figure 6.2. The different volumes correspond to diameters with 1 cm increments between them. The relationships appear linear and parallel in a log–probit scale, if very small tumours are excluded since their measurement is particularly imprecise. The estimated slopes of the two regression lines are 0.45 (95% CI: 0.40–0.49) for metastases detectable at diagnosis and 0.41 (95% CI: 0.34–0.49) for metastases at 20 years, and are not significantly different ($p = 0.50$). Consequently, the hypothesis of an exponential growth pattern is not rejected on the basis of these data.

With the Gompertzian growth model, the slopes of the two relationships are expected to be different, since the slope representing the relationship between the tumour size and the proportion of metastases at diagnosis is steeper than that of the relationship between the tumour size and metastases in the long term. The two curves are expected to intersect at a point corresponding to the plateau of the tumour growth curve. This is not however what we observe (Figure 6.2).

If we assume that

1. almost all metastases are present at the time of diagnosis, i.e. initiated before treatment, and become detectable within 20 years, and that

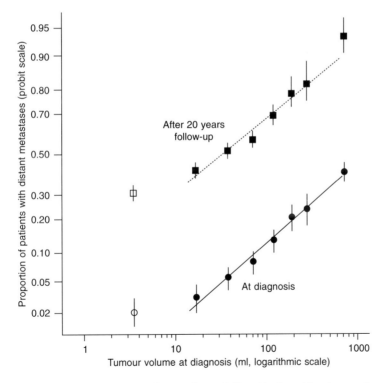

Figure 6.2 Relationship between tumour volume at diagnosis (logarithmic scale) and proportion of patients with distant metastases at diagnosis (● ○), and after 20 years of follow-up (■ □) (probit scale). The volumes correspond to clinical tumour diameters which are midpoints of classes in Table 1. Data corresponding to very small tumours (empty symbols) are not included in the computation of the regression lines because the estimation of the tumour size is not sufficiently accurate. The slopes of the two regression lines are not significantly different

2. no metastasis can be initiated after complete local treatment,

we can then estimate the median tumour *volume at metastasis initiation*, as the tumour volume at diagnosis corresponding to a 50% *probability of metastases in the long term*. This estimation was performed using the SAS PROC PROBIT procedure and was found to be equal to 31 ml (95% confidence interval (CI): 25–38 ml). Similarly, the median tumour *volume at metastasis detection* can be estimated as the tumour volume at diagnosis corresponding to a 50% *probability of metastasis at diagnosis* and is equal to 1251 ml (95% CI: 939–1668 ml).

6.3.2 Relationship between the proportion of patients with metastases at diagnosis (p_a) and the cumulative proportion of patients with metastases after 20 years of follow-up (p_b)

The relationship between the probability of metastasis at diagnosis and the probability of metastasis after 20 years of follow-up in groups of patients defined according to the size of the tumour, is linear in a probit–probit co-ordinate system (Figure 6.3). The slope

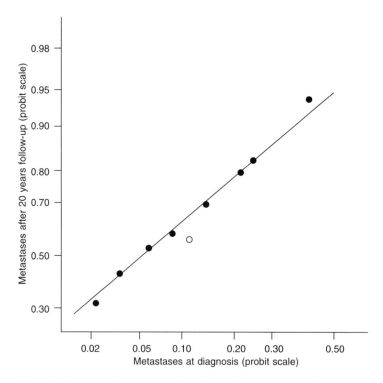

Figure 6.3 Relationship between the proportion of patients with metastases at diagnosis (probit scale) and the cumulative proportion of patients with metastases after 20 years of follow-up (probit scale). Full symbols correspond to groups of patients defined according to the size of the tumour, the empty symbol represents the overall population of patients. A linear regression line with slope 1 fits the data points. All the groups, including very small tumours, lie along this regression line

(1.07, 95% CI: 1.00–1.14) is not significantly different from 1, which is to be expected, based on the hypothesis of exponential growth. Let us assume that the slope is indeed equal to 1. Then the relationship between p_a and p_b is:

$$\Phi^{-1}(p_a) = \Phi^{-1}(p_b) - \delta$$

where Φ^{-1} is the probit transformation. To estimate the value of the constant δ one can average the differences $\Phi^{-1}(p_b) - \Phi^{-1}(p_a)$ over the eight classes of tumour volumes. This leads to

$$\delta = 1.62 \quad (95\% \text{ CI: } 1.49–1.75)$$

For the overall population (last line in Table 6.1):

$$\Phi^{-1}(p_b) - \Phi^{-1}(p_a) = \Phi^{-1}(0.56) - \Phi^{-1}(0.11) = 1.38$$

which is outside the 95% CI estimated from groups defined according to the size of the tumour. This discrepancy is explained by the fact that δ depends on both the standard deviation of the log tumour volume at metastasis initiation $\sqrt{\text{Var}(\log V_{0i})}$ and at tumour diagnosis $\sqrt{\text{Var}(\log V_{di})}$ (see appendix, relations B.5 and B.10). $\sqrt{\text{Var}(\log V_{di})}$ is larger in the overall population than in groups of patients defined on the basis of the tumour size at treatment. The values of $\sqrt{\text{Var}(\log V_{di})}$ are directly estimable from our data. When $\sqrt{\text{Var}(\log V_{di})}$ is taken into account, a correct δ value is estimated for the overall population, leading to appropriate predictions of the proportions of patients with metastases in the long term. In groups of patients defined according to tumour size, $\sqrt{\text{Var}(\log V_{di})}$ is too small to change the estimation of delta and consequently the predictions of the proportions of patients with metastases.

The proportion of patients with metastases in the long term can be predicted by adding either 1.62 or 1.38 to the probit of the proportion of patients with metastasis (Table 6.1). The addition of 1.62 leads to a satisfactory fit for each group of patients defined on the basis of the tumour size at treatment, but not for the total population, for which the value 1.38 must be added to obtain a satisfactory fit. The use of 1.38 instead of 1.62 is justified by the necessity to take into account the greater variability of the overall population compared to the groups of patients defined as a function of tumour volume.

6.4 Discussion

In the various groups of patients studied, the cumulative proportion of patients with metastases in the long term is strongly related to the proportion of patients with metastases at diagnosis. This relationship can be explained by a simple model of the natural history of breast cancer, assuming that tumour growth is exponential and that the occurrence of metastases is determined in relation to the timing of tumour treatment.

The relationship established above is based on data on patients with newly diagnosed invasive breast cancers who did not receive adjuvant chemotherapy. The patients were not selected according to their metastasis status and were evaluated for the presence of distant metastases with standard procedures. This model, therefore, cannot be used to estimate the long-term probability of metastasis in a population of patients receiving adjuvant therapies. Such estimation will become possible as long-term follow-up (of the order of 20 years) becomes available on large numbers of patients treated in the era of adjuvant therapy.

The co-ordinate systems (log–probit or probit–probit) we used are rarely used in studies investigating prognostic factors. In a classic co-ordinate system (log–linear), the relationship between the logarithm of the tumour volume at diagnosis and the long-term probability of metastases can be considered as linear (Figure 6.4). In fact, with probabilities ranging from 20% to 80%, it is difficult to distinguish between the log–linear and the log–probit models. However, the linearity does not hold for the relation between the logarithm of the tumour volume and the probability of metastasis at diagnosis (Figure 6.4). A logistic analysis would have been adequate for the description of the relationships between tumour volume and probability of metastases. Moreover, the logistic and probit relationships are not distinguishable in the range of probabilities considered in this paper. However, the probit approach permits a direct transition to reasoning in terms of volume at initiation or at detection of metastases. Therefore, the probit relationship was used.

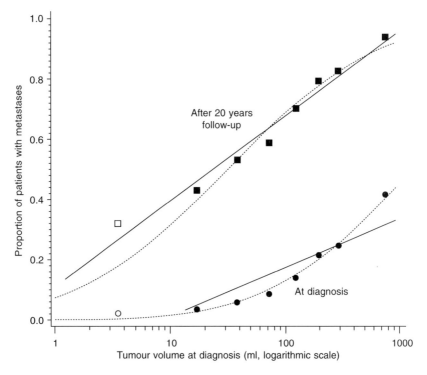

Figure 6.4 Relationship between tumour volume at diagnosis (logarithmic scale) and the proportion of patients with distant metastases at diagnosis, and after 20 years of follow-up. The solid lines correspond to linear regressions of the proportion of patients with metastases on the logarithm of the tumour volume at diagnosis (log–linear model). The dotted lines correspond to the linear regression of probit of the proportion of patients with metastases on the logarithm of the tumour volume at diagnosis (log–probit model). The log–linear model adequately fits the data corresponding to metastases after 20 years of follow-up but does not fit the data for metastasis at diagnosis. The log–probit model is acceptable both for metastases after 20 years of follow-up and for metastasis at diagnosis

The simplest way to deal with the relationship observed is to consider that the volume of the primary tumour is multiplied by a constant value during the growth of metastases (which takes place between the initiation and detection of the metastases). Graphically, this means that the horizontal distance between the curves linking the proportion of patients with metastases in the long term and at diagnosis and the tumour volume at diagnosis is constant (Figure 6.1). The constancy of the ratio between the tumour volume at the detection of metastases and at the initiation of metastases is a consequence of assuming exponential growth both for the tumour and for the metastases, and of proportionality between the growth rates of tumours and those of metastases (constant ratio between the growth rate of a tumour and of its metastases).

Our results are at variance with the general opinion that tumours exhibit a Gompertzian growth pattern. This opinion is based on experimental data on tumour growth in animals, in which growth rates decrease when the tumours become large. With the Gompertzian growth pattern, this slowing down is supposed to take place throughout tumour growth. This phenomenon was not evident in our data. This does not seem to be due to a lack of power. Let us make an analogy with animal experiments. The volume of the tumour $V(t)$ is measured once, at time t after implantation in each animal. The tumour implantation procedure is standardised and the initial tumour volume V_0 is assumed to be the same for all tumours. In this manner, V_0, $V(t)$ and the time t^* between V_0 and V_1 are known for each animal. With our model, the V_0 and V_1 distributions are known, as well as t^* (with the duration of growth of metastases being used as a time scale). Our indirect estimates of the parameters of the distributions of V_0 and V_1 are as precise as direct measurements performed on at least two thousand tumours. This analogy with experiments involving at most a few hundred animals leads to the conclusion that our indirect estimation of the growth pattern is more precise than most estimates based on experimental data. The apparent contradiction between our results and experimental data can be resolved by considering other simple growth models. For example, a logistic growth pattern is compatible with our result (a prolonged phase of exponential growth) and with experimental data (a phase of retardation), and fits experimental data just as well as the Gompertzian model (Gratton et al., 1978).

There are no data concerning the relationship between tumour and metastasis doubling times, and the hypothesis of proportionality between tumour and metastasis doubling times cannot be verified. We chose it because of its simplicity. If a Gompertzian growth pattern is assumed, it can be demonstrated that the relationship observed between the proportion of patients with metastases at diagnosis and the cumulative proportion of patients with metastases in the long term implies that the ratio between the doubling time of the tumour and its metastases varies as a function of the tumour volume at the time of metastatic dissemination.

A major practical application of this work is the possibility of use of the proportion of patients with metastases at diagnosis as a surrogate endpoint for screening. Long-term follow-up is required for classical evaluation based on mortality and various sources of bias such as lead time bias (Zelen and Feinleib, 1969) and length bias (Feinleib and Zelen, 1969) should be taken into account in such an evaluation strategy. Various surrogate endpoints have been proposed, including the proportion of tumours with advanced stages (stage II or more) at diagnosis, or the proportion of patients with axillary metastases at diagnosis, but these surrogates are not necessarily directly linked to the proportion of patients who will be cured. The advantage gained with the proportion of patients with detectable metastases at diagnosis (distant disease in the AJC classification, stage IV in the TNM classification) is that they can be identified immediately and there is no need to follow up the population for many years. Of course frank clinical metastases at diagnosis will be very rare in a population exposed to mammographic screening and an evaluation based on clinical metastases would require large numbers of cases in total to contain a small number of metastatic cases. The above-mentioned biases are arguably avoided when using the proportion of patients with metastases at diagnosis because there is a 'structural' relationship between this proportion and the proportion of patients who will eventually be cured. As the relationship between the proportion of patients with metastases at diagnosis and the subsequent mortality in the whole population has been established, the former may be used instead of mortality as an endpoint in evaluation of screening programmes for breast cancer.

The relation between the proportion of patients with metastases at diagnosis and the proportion in the long term is slightly different in subgroups of patients to that observed in the total case population. This discrepancy is explained by the importance of variability. Population characteristics are not only described by the mean; to make valid extrapolations, this problem of variability should be taken into account. In practice this is not always feasible but we can make informed comparisons between populations using the proportions of patients with metastases at diagnosis, assuming equal variability.

As the proportion of patients with metastasis at diagnosis is usually very small, the accuracy of this indicator might seem questionable. Let us consider a population in which screening is proposed with the aim of reducing long-term breast cancer mortality from 40% to 30%, assuming that long-term breast cancer mortality is exclusively caused by metastases. The number of breast cancer patients needed to demonstrate this 10% reduction in mortality is equal to 900 (Machin and Campbell, 1987) (log rank test, two-sided $\alpha = 0.05$, $\beta = 0.10$). This is the minimum number required based on the hypothesis that no patients are lost to follow-up. More than 15 years will be needed to obtain the result. In contrast, according to our model, this reduction in long-term mortality is equivalent to a reduction from 5.1% to 2.8% in the proportion of patients with metastases at diagnosis. Approximately 3100 patients with breast cancers will therefore be needed to demonstrate (Friedman et al., 1985) such a reduction ($\alpha = 0.05$, $\beta = 0.10$), but in this case, the answer will be immediate.

6.5 Conclusion

Patients with detectable metastases can be viewed as the visible part of an iceberg. Knowing the proportion of patients with metastases at diagnosis is sufficient to estimate the proportion of patients who will be cured, just as knowing the size of the visible part of an iceberg makes it possible to evaluate the whole iceberg.

References

Collins, V.P., Loeffler, K.R. and Tivey, H. (1956). Observations on the growth rates of human tumours. Am. J. Roentgen, **76**, 988–1000.
Feinleib, M. and Zelen, M. (1969). Some pitfalls in the evaluation of screening programs. Arch. Environ. Health, **19**, 412–15.

Finney, D.J. (1964). *Statistical Methods in Biological Assay* (2nd edition). Charles Griffin, London.

Friedman, L.M., Furberg, C.D. and DeMets, D.L. (1985). *Fundamentals of Clinical Trials*. PSG Publishing Co., Littleton.

Gratton, R.J., Appleton, D.R. and Alwiswasy, M.K. (1978). The measurement of tumour growth rates. In: Valleron, A.-J. and Macdonald, P.D.M. (eds), *Biomathematics and Cell Kinetics*. Elsevier/North-Holland, Amsterdam: pp. 325–32.

Koscielny, S., Tubiana, M., Lê, M.G., Valleron, A.-J., Mouriesse, H., Contesso, G. *et al.* (1984). Breast cancer: Relationship between the size of the primary tumour and the probability of metastatic dissemination. *Br. J. Cancer*, **49**, 709–15.

Lacour, J., Juret, P. and Sarrazin, D. (1968). Protocole schématique de traitement des cancers du sein à l'Institut Gustave Roussy. *Rev. Prat. (Paris)*, **18**, 3595.

Machin, D. and Campbell, M.J. (1987). *Statistical Tables for the Design of Clinical Trials*. Blackwell Scientific Publications, Oxford.

Zelen, M. and Feinleib, M. (1969). On the theory of screening for chronic diseases. *Biometrika*, **56**, 601–14.

Appendix A: Relationship between the tumour volume at initiation and detection of metastasis

Let us consider the evolution of a primary tumour for individual i (Figure 6.5). Two main events will occur if this tumour is left untreated: the initiation of the first metastasis when the tumour reaches volume V_{0i} and the detection of the metastasis when it reaches volume V_{1i}. If the tumour is treated, there are three possibilities which are dependent on the tumour volume at the first treatment V_{di} compared to V_{0i} and V_{1i}:

1. V_{di} is smaller than V_{0i}; in this case, local treatment prevents the initiation of the metastasis and cures the tumour.
2. V_{di} is larger than volume V_{0i} but smaller than V_{1i}, i.e. metastases have been initiated but are not yet detectable; in this case the local tumour is cured by local treatment but metastases will appear later during the follow-up.
3. V_{di} is larger than volume V_{1i}; here remote metastases are already detectable at the time of treatment.

The simplest hypothesis concerning tumours and the growth of metastases is an exponential growth pattern (Collins *et al.*, 1956) for the primary tumour and for the metastases, with proportionality between metastasis and tumour doubling times. Based on this hypothesis, relationships have been established between the volume of the primary tumour at the initiation and detection of metastases.

Let t_i be the time elapsed between tumour volumes V_{0i} and V_{1i}. This time corresponds to the duration of growth of metastases from initiation to detection,

$$\frac{t_i}{\log V_{1i} - \log V_{0i}} = \frac{DTV_i}{\log 2} \tag{A.1}$$

where DTV_i is the doubling time of the tumour for individual i.

During the same time t_i, the volume of the metastases grows from W_{0i}, volume of the metastasis at initiation (~1 clonogenic cell) to W_{1i}, volume of the metastasis at detection (~1 ml), and

$$\frac{t_i}{\log W_{1i} - \log W_{0i}} = \frac{DTW_i}{\log 2} \tag{A.2}$$

where DTW_i is the metastases doubling time. The volumes of the metastases at initiation W_{0i} and at detection W_{1i} are assumed to be equal for all individuals, therefore

$$t_i = \frac{k\,DTW_i}{\log 2} \tag{A.3}$$

where k is a constant. If DTV_i and DTW_i are proportional, from (A.1) and (A.3),

$$\log V_{1i} - \log V_{0i} = \frac{k\,DTW_i}{DTV_i} = k' \tag{A.4}$$

Therefore, based on the hypotheses of (A.1) exponential growth patterns for the primary tumour and the metastases, (A.2) constancy across individuals for both the volume of the metastasis at the time of initiation and for the volume of the metastasis at the time of detection and (A.3) proportionality between metastasis and tumour doubling times, the

(a) First treatment before metastasis initiation ($V_d < V_0$)

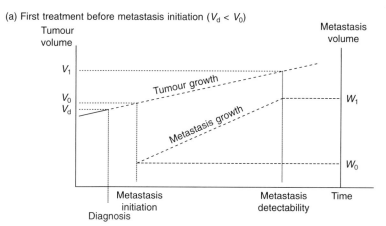

(b) First treatment between metastasis initiation and met. detectability ($V_0 < V_d < V_1$)

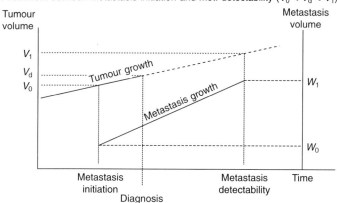

(c) First treatment when metastases are detectable ($V_d > V_1$)

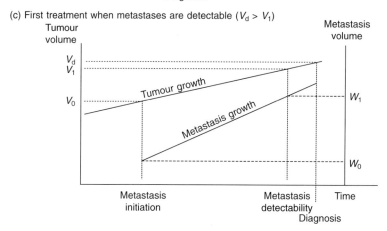

Figure 6.5 Tumour volume and volume of metastases as a function of time, for
(a) first treatment before the initiation of metastasis
(b) first treatment between the initiation and detection of metastasis and
(c) first treatment when metastases are detectable

difference $\log V_{1i} - \log V_{0i}$ is constant. This leads to the following relations for the expectation (E) and the variance Var of the distribution of the logarithm of tumour volume at metastases detection:

$$E(\log V_{1i}) = E(\log V_{0i}) + k' \tag{A.5}$$

$$\mathrm{Var}(\log V_{1i}) = \mathrm{Var}(\log V_{0i}) \tag{A.6}$$

The expectation and variance of $\log V_{0i}$ and $\log V_{1i}$ can be indirectly estimated according to the methods described by Finney (1964). For this purpose, the relationship between the tumour volume at treatment and the probability of metastasis at diagnosis for this volume is linearised in a log–probit co-ordinate system. The same method is used to linearise the relationship between the tumour volume at treatment and the long-term probability of metastasis for this volume. The values of $\sqrt{\mathrm{Var}(\log V_{0i})}$ and $\sqrt{\mathrm{Var}(\log V_{1i})}$ are equal to the inverse of the slopes. Based on the above three hypotheses, these values are equal and the two lines are parallel. Non-parallelism of these two lines would lead to a global rejection of the three hypotheses.

By relaxing the hypothesis of exponential growth, and selecting a Gompertzian growth model, the following relationships are obtained (Gratton *et al.*, 1978):

$$E(\log V_{0i}) = [E(\log V_{1i}) + (R - 1) \log V_\infty]/R \tag{A.7}$$

$$\sqrt{\mathrm{Var}(\log V_{0i})} = \sqrt{\mathrm{Var}(\log V_{1i})}/R \tag{A.8}$$

where R is a function of t, the time since initiation of metastases. The tumour volume corresponding to the plateau of the growth curve V_∞ is equal to:

$$V_\infty = \exp\left\{ \frac{R\,E(\log V_{1i}) - E(\log V_{0i})}{R - 1} \right\} \tag{A.9}$$

and corresponds to the point where the two log–probit curves meet.

Appendix B: Relationship between the probability of metastases at diagnosis and the probability of metastases in the long term

Let x_i be an indicator of the 'size' of the tumour at the time of diagnosis, expressed as the position of $\log V_{di}$ with respect to $\log V_{1i}$ and $\log V_{0i}$:

$$x_i = \frac{\log V_{di} - \log V_{0i}}{\log V_{1i} - \log V_{0i}} = \frac{\log V_{di} - \log V_{0i}}{k'} \tag{B.1}$$

When $\log V_{di} = \log V_{0i}$, i.e. when the diagnosis is at the time of the initiation of metastasis, x takes the value 0. When $\log V_{di} = \log V_{1i}$, i.e. when the diagnosis is made upon detection of metastasis, x takes the value 1. Values of x between 0 and 1 correspond to tumours diagnosed while subclinical metastases are present.

The probability of metastases being detectable at diagnosis p_a is equal to

$$p_a = p(x \geq 1) \tag{B.2}$$

and the probability of metastases occurring in the long term p_b is equal to

$$p_b = p(x \geq 0) \tag{B.3}$$

The relationship between these probabilities is governed by the distribution of x

$$E(x) = [E(\log V_{di}) - E(\log V_{0i})]/k' \tag{B.4}$$

$$\text{Var } x = [\text{Var}(\log V_{di}) + \text{Var}(\log V_{0i})]/k'^2 \tag{B.5}$$

As the distributions of $\log V_{di}$ and $\log V_{0i}$ are both approximately normal, x can be considered as normally distributed, and $x' = (x - E(x))/\sqrt{\text{Var } x}$, has a standard normal distribution whose cumulative distribution function is Φ, hence

$$1 - p_b = \Phi(-E(x)/\sqrt{\text{Var } x}) \tag{B.6}$$

$$1 - p_a = \Phi([1 - E(x)]/\sqrt{\text{Var } x}) \tag{B.7}$$

This leads to

$$\Phi^{-1}(1 - p_b) = -E(x)/\sqrt{\text{Var } x} \tag{B.8}$$

and to

$$\Phi^{-1}(1 - p_a) = [1 - E(x)]/\sqrt{\text{Var } x} \tag{B.9}$$

The transformation Φ^{-1} is the probit. From (B.8) and (B.9), the following relation is obtained:

$$\Phi^{-1}(1 - p_a) = 1/\sqrt{\text{Var } x} + \Phi^{-1}(1 - p_b) \tag{B.10}$$

which depends on both $\sqrt{\text{Var}(\log V_{0i})}$ and $\sqrt{\text{Var}(\log V_{di})}$ as shown in equation (B.5). In groups of patients defined according to the size of the tumour at diagnosis, the variability of the tumour volume at diagnosis is negligible as compared to the variability of the tumour volume at the initiation of metastases. Therefore $\sqrt{\text{Var } x}$ is approximately equal to $\sqrt{\text{Var}(\log V_{0i})}/k'$. In the overall population, $\sqrt{\text{Var}(\log V_{di})}$ is no longer negligible and $\sqrt{\text{Var } x}$ is underestimated if $\sqrt{\text{Var}(\log V_{0i})}/k'$ is used as an estimator.

7

Use of an illness–death model to predict the effects of different breast screening intervals

Hsiu-Hsi Chen, Ming-Fang Yen and Laszlo Tabar

7.1 Introduction

In screening for breast cancer, it is of interest from a cost-effectiveness point of view to estimate the relative benefits of different interscreening intervals. Clearly, a shorter interscreening interval would lead to more cancers being detected early by screening, and *potentially* to more lives being saved. A very short interval (e.g. less than one year), however, would probably be unacceptable to the target population and would in any case be prohibitively expensive. International variation in intervals used tends to range from one year to three years (Shapiro *et al.*, 1998).

In this chapter we estimate rates of development of preclinical breast cancer, progression from preclinical to clinical disease and progression from clinical disease to death from breast cancer. These are used in turn to simulate screening regimes of varying intervals, and to estimate the mortality reductions likely to accrue from the different intervals.

7.2 Data

The data used are from the control group of the Swedish Two-County Trial (Tabar *et al.*, 2000) of mammographic screening for breast cancer, in the age groups 50–59 and 60–69 at the time of randomisation. These groups comprised 16 805 and 16 269 women respectively. During the screening phase of the trial, lasting approximately eight years, the control women were not invited to screening, except for a single screen at the close of this phase. Of the women alive and free of breast cancer at this time, 14 479 (87% attendance) in the 50–59 age group, and 12 778 (80% attendance) women in the 60–69 age group attended for screening.

During the screening phase, there were 221 breast cancers diagnosed clinically and 94 screen-detected at the single screen at the close of the trial in the 50–59 age group. Because registration details of one of the clinical cancers were not available in time for analysis, only 220 of these cancers were used in the analysis. The corresponding figures for the 60–69 age group were 277 clinical and 140 screen-detected tumours. There were 97 breast cancer deaths to 31 December 1996 among the clinically detected tumours in the 50–59 age group and 112 deaths in the 60–69 age group.

7.3 Model and methods

We used the data described above to estimate rates of progression between the following states:

State 0: no detectable breast cancer
State 1: preclinical screen-detectable breast cancer
State 2: clinical (symptomatic) breast cancer
State 3: death from breast cancer

We assume that progression occurs as a Markov process (Cox and Miller, 1965) with the following matrix of instantaneous transition rates

$$\begin{pmatrix} -\lambda_1 & \lambda_1 & 0 & 0 \\ 0 & -\lambda_2 & \lambda_2 & 0 \\ 0 & 0 & -\lambda_3 & \lambda_3 \\ 0 & 0 & 0 & 0 \end{pmatrix}$$

This means that the probability of moving from state 0 (no detectable disease) to state 1 (preclinical breast cancer) in a very short time δt is $\lambda_1 \delta t$. The corresponding probabilities of transition from state 1 to state 2 and state 2 to state 3 are $\lambda_2 \delta t$ and $\lambda_3 \delta t$.

   Implicit in the above are various assumptions. Firstly, no reversal of disease is possible; secondly, an individual cannot cross two state barriers at the same instant. The latter means that it is not possible to progress from no detectable disease to clinical disease without spending some time, however short, in the preclinical disease state. By the same assumption, one cannot progress directly from preclinical breast cancer to death from breast cancer without at least some period of clinical symptomatic disease. Finally, the Markov chain model implies that if an individual is in state i ($i = 0, 1, 2$) at a given time T, the probability of progressing to state $i + 1$ within a subsequent specified time interval of length t is

$$1 - e^{-\lambda_{i+1} t}$$

This probability is independent of that individual's history before time T.

   From the above instantaneous transition rate matrix, the corresponding matrix of finite time transition probabilities can be calculated by standard algebraic methods as

$$\begin{pmatrix} P_{00}(t) & P_{01}(t) & P_{02}(t) & P_{03}(t) \\ 0 & P_{11}(t) & P_{12}(t) & P_{13}(t) \\ 0 & 0 & P_{22}(t) & P_{23}(t) \\ 0 & 0 & 0 & 1 \end{pmatrix}$$

In the above, $P_{ij}(t)$ is the probability of an individual's being in state j at time $T + t$ given that the individual was in state i at time T; T and t are any non-negative real numbers. $P_{ij}(t)$ is a combination of exponential functions of the λ_j ($j = 1, 2, 3$) and t. For further details, see Chapter 5.

Combination of these probabilities with the data were used to construct the likelihood function. For example, for the age group 50–59, the likelihood function is

$$L = (P_{00}(m)P_{00}(8)/(P_{00}(m) + P_{01}(m)))^{14385} \times ((P_{00}(m)P_{01}(8)$$

$$+ P_{01}(m)P_{11}(8))/(P_{00}(m) + P_{01}(m)))^{94} \times \prod_{k=1}^{220} \{(P_{00}(m)P_{00}(t_k - \delta t)P_{02}(\delta t)$$

$$+ P_{00}(m)P_{01}(t_k - \delta t)P_{12}(\delta t) + P_{01}(m)P_{11}(t_k - \delta t)P_{12}(\delta t))/(P_{00}(m)$$

$$+ P_{01}(m))\} \times \prod_{l=1}^{97} P_{22}(s_l - \delta t)P_{23}(\delta t)$$

where m is the average age at randomisation (55 years in this case), t_k ($k = 1, 2, ..., 220$) are times from randomisation to diagnosis of clinical cancer, δt represents a very short time (in this case, one month) and s_l ($l = 1, 2, ..., 97$) are times from diagnosis of clinical cancer to death from breast cancer. The division by $(P_{00}(m) + P_{01}(m))$ is to condition on the fact that in this study, all women with clinical breast cancer prior to randomisation were excluded.

Since the likelihood function and its logarithm were long and complex, the above was used to calculate the expected number of transitions of each type. We then generated a series of equations for estimation, of the form:

Observed outcomes = expected outcomes + error

This series of equations was solved as a non-linear regression, as described in Chapter 5.

The above yielded estimates of λ_1, λ_2 and λ_3. These were then used to simulate, for each age group, a female population of size 10 000 over a six-year period, with annual, two-yearly and three-yearly screening, and as a control population no screening except for a single screen at the end of the six-year period. These in turn gave the numbers of screen-detected cancer, clinical cancers and using λ_3, the expected 10-year deaths from the latter, diagnosed under the four regimes. Deaths from the preclinical screen-detected cancers were estimated from the 10-year case fatality rate observed for the screen-detected tumours in the Two-County Trial. From these, we calculated the expected deaths from breast cancer for each regime and the relative risks for the three screening regimes compared to the control.

7.4 Results

Table 7.1 shows the estimates of the transition rates and 95% confidence intervals on these. As one might expect, the λ_1's are roughly equal to the incidence rates in the two age groups within the trial (Tabar et al., 1992). The λ_3's can be translated to case fatality rates for clinical cancers. For the 50–59 age group, the 10-year fatality rate (breast cancer deaths only) is calculated as $1 - e^{-10 \times 0.0361} = 0.303$, i.e. 30.3% fatality. The corresponding

Table 7.1 Estimated transition rates and 95% confidence intervals by age

Age group	Transition	Estimated rate	95% confidence interval
50–59	No disease to preclinical	0.0019	0.0018–0.0020
	Preclinical to clinical	0.2920	0.2795–0.3045
	Clinical to death	0.0361	0.0347–0.0375
60–69	No disease to preclinical	0.0027	0.0026–0.0028
	Preclinical to clinical	0.2454	0.2356–0.2553
	Clinical to death	0.0324	0.0310–0.0338

Table 7.2 Predicted 10-year breast cancer deaths in populations of size 16 000 from tumours diagnosed over a six-year period, for various screening intervals: results of simulation using the estimates in Table 7.1

Age group	Screening regime	Predicted deaths in screened group	Predicted deaths in control group	Predicted relative risk
50–59	Annual	29.53	54.36	0.54
	Two-yearly	32.68	54.36	0.60
	Three-yearly	35.27	54.36	0.65
60–69	Annual	40.24	72.79	0.55
	Two-yearly	43.60	72.79	0.60
	Three-yearly	46.22	72.79	0.63

figure for the 60–69 age group is 27.7%. These compare to 10-year death rates for screen-detected cases of 9.8% and 8.6%.

Results of simulations are shown in Table 7.2. The results predict reductions in breast cancer mortality of 46%, 40% and 35% from, respectively, annual, two-yearly and three-yearly screening in women aged 50–59. For women aged 60–69, the expected mortality reductions are 45%, 40% and 37%. This means that in the 50–59 age group, annual screening would confer a relative breast cancer mortality reduction of 16% over three-yearly screening, and an absolute reduction of 11% over three-yearly screening. For the 60–69 age group, annual screening is predicted to confer a further relative reduction of 13% and an absolute reduction of 8% over three-yearly screening.

7.5 Discussion

The above results involve various assumptions, possibly the strongest of which is that probabilities of future progression given the current state are independent of past history, which is an implication of the homogeneous Markov chain model. This is probably a reasonable approximation for the age groups considered here, but in younger women, there may be heterogeneity ('frailties' in statistical terms) which render this assumption unsafe (Chen *et al.*, 1998). Also, for each age group, the preclinical incidence rate for that age group is assumed constant throughout past life up to that age group. This is clearly untrue, but our previous work (Tabar *et al.*, 1995), and indeed the estimates of λ_1 here, show that estimation is robust to this failure, and that estimates corresponding to the known incidence for the age group under consideration usually result.

The formal modelling approach has the advantage that predicted effects of different screening regimes are based on empirical estimates of disease incidence, progression and fatality from a unified analysis of real data. The inclusion of progression to death in the model is a technical advance on our previous work (Chen *et al.*, 1997). The results are consistent with the previous finding that the interval between screens becomes less crucial for older populations. The predicted mortality results are also consistent with those observed in the Two-County Trial. Our estimation and simulation procedure above predicted for three-yearly screening a 35% mortality reduction in the 50–59 age group and a 37% reduction in the 60–69 age group. The reductions actually observed were 34% and 40%, respectively (Tabar *et al.*, 1995).

References

Chen, H.H., Duffy, S.W., Tabar, L. and Day, N.E. (1997). Markov chain models for progression of breast cancer, Part 1: Tumour attributes and the preclinical detectable phase. *Journal of Epidemiology and Biostatistics*, **2**, 9–23.

Chen, H.H., Duffy, S.W., Tabar, L. and Day, N.E. (1998). Authors' reply. *Journal of Epidemiology and Biostatistics*, **3**, 424–7.

Cox, D.R. and Miller, H.D. (1965). *The Theory of Stochastic Processes*. Methuen, London.

Shapiro, S., Coleman, E.A., Broeders, M. *et al.* (1998). Breast cancer screening programmes in 22 countries: current policies, administration and guidelines. *International Journal of Epidemiology*, **27**, 735–42.

Tabar, L., Fagerberg, G., Duffy, S.W., Day, N.E., Gad, A. and Grontoft, O. (1992). Update of the Swedish Two-County program of mammographic screening for breast cancer. *Radiologic Clinics of North America*, **30**, 187–210.

Tabar, L., Fagerberg, G., Chen, H.H., Duffy, S.W., Smart, C.R., Gad, A. and Smith, R.A. (1995). Efficacy of breast cancer screening by age: new results from the Swedish Two-County Trial. *Cancer*, **75**, 2507–17.

Tabar, L., Vitak, B., Chen, H.H., Duffy, S.W., Yen, M.F., Chiang, C.F., Krusemo, U.B., Tot, T. and Smith, R.A. (2000). The Swedish Two-County Trial twenty years later: updated mortality results and new insights from long-term follow-up. *Radiologic Clinics of North America*, **38**, 625–51.

8

Screening evaluation and monitoring: some practical considerations

Jenny McCann and Diane Stockton

The decision to implement screening nationally in the UK was based on firm evidence from randomised controlled trials which showed that breast cancer screening could significantly reduce breast cancer mortality. The report from a working party chaired by Professor Sir Patrick Forrest recommended the introduction of a national breast cancer screening programme (Forrest, 1986) based on the design of the successful Swedish Two-County Study which achieved a 35% reduction in mortality in women in the target age range (Tabar *et al.*, 1985, 1987).

Following the introduction of any screening programme, rigorous monitoring and evaluation of programme performance and impact are essential in order to ensure that the programme functions optimally and achieves its goal of reducing the burden of disease in the target population. Clearly mortality reduction is the ultimate goal of cancer screening. However, in the Swedish Two-County Study there was a seven-year delay from randomisation (virtually contemporaneous with first screening invitation in the study group) before a significant reduction in breast cancer deaths could be observed (Day *et al.*, 1989). If a service screening programme is introduced in a region in a staggered fashion, the delay before a mortality reduction is observed may be longer. Interim measures of programme effectiveness are required in order to determine whether the programme is on course for delivering the expected benefit. Such information may be used to implement remedial intervention if a programme is found not to be performing as expected.

Population screening for breast cancer was introduced in East Anglia in 1989. Following national guidelines, women aged 50–64 are offered screening by mammography at three-year intervals. The approach taken to the evaluation of its effectiveness was based on the principle outlined by Day *et al.* (1989) that mortality reduction is achieved through a logical sequence of events which starts with acceptance of the invitation for screening:

1. compliance at first screen;
2. detection of many small lesions at that screen;
3. low incidence of interval cancers in women screened negative;
4. effective detection of many small lesions at second screen;
5. reduction in incidence rate of advanced cancers in the invited population; and
6. reduction in mortality.

This sequence of events provides the programme evaluator with a number of more short-term outcomes which must be achieved if the programme is to achieve its aim. These include good compliance, high detection rate for small invasive cancers at prevalence screen, low rate of interval cancers following this first screen, high detection rate of small cancers at second screen and a reduction in incidence of advanced (for example stage II or above) cancers (Day *et al.*, 1989). This latter has been shown to be very strongly predictive of the subsequent reduction in mortality (Tabar *et al.*, 1985; Day *et al.*, 1989). Note that it is *incidence* of advanced tumours in the invited population which has this predictive power, and not the *proportion* of advanced tumours in the cancers diagnosed. The latter is subject to length bias, whereby the more indolent tumours are more likely to be detected at screening, which in turn gives an artificially higher proportion of less advanced tumours, and therefore an artificially lower proportion of more advanced, in the invited population.

The theory behind screening programme evaluation has been more than adequately described elsewhere (Day *et al.*, 1989; Hennekens and Buring, 1987; Day, 1996). The aim of this chapter is to describe some of the practical issues and problems which we have encountered and addressed whilst monitoring and evaluating the screening programme in East Anglia.

8.2 Information requirements

The evaluation of screening requires access to information systems that permit monitoring of the interim indicators outlined in the pathway above. These will include:

- mechanisms for identifying all cases of breast cancer arising in the target population;
- detailed information on the pathology of these cancers;
- means of determining how all cancers arising in the target population were detected (e.g. screen detected, interval cancer, etc.).

Furthermore, if the evaluation is to be meaningful, further data are required regarding a

- suitable unscreened comparison group.

8.3 Choice of comparison group

Options for selecting a comparison group against which to measure the effect of screening include (1) using a historical cohort from a period before screening was implemented, (2) using a geographically neighbouring unscreened group and (3) comparing screened with unscreened women. The first of these requires availability of reliable incidence and prognostic indicator data. Problems associated with this approach include the possibility of changes in incidence and prognostic indicators taking place independently of screening over time (McCann *et al.*, 1998).

These problems are reduced in the second option: choosing a control group of as yet uninvited women, who should be similar in every way to the invited group except that they have not yet received the invitation to screening. Clearly this is only practical if screening is introduced in a staggered fashion in the area of interest and if sufficient cases arise in each age group of interest before screening is introduced. This group has the advantage of providing a contemporaneous group who are more likely to be subject to the same potential influences on breast cancer incidence (e.g. age at menopause, HRT/oral contraceptive use, etc.) and the same level of clinical work-up and care (e.g. axillary node investigation and type of surgery) as the invited group. This then provides an unbiased data set for comparison.

The last of the options – comparing screened with unscreened women – is to be avoided. This is because for the rigorous evaluation of a screening programme, one should compare the *whole* of the invited population (which will contain, among it, those who would refuse an invitation for screening) with a similar, but uninvited, population to avoid selection bias. The latter may arise because people who are more health-conscious and therefore potentially more healthy *a priori* are more likely to participate in a screening programme.

The need for care in the choice of comparison group and the relative disadvantages and limitations of each of these options have been discussed more fully elsewhere (Day *et al.*, 1989; Duffy *et al.*, 1991; Day, 1996). The quality of the data for the comparison group against which the effects of screening are evaluated is of paramount importance and the need for rigour in establishing this baseline cannot be stressed too highly. In East Anglia, we have used both a historical cohort and a contemporaneous, not-yet-invited group to provide baseline information against which to measure the effectiveness of screening (McCann *et al.*, 1998). Figure 8.1 shows the variation in estimated underlying incidence of advanced breast cancer, against which incidence in the invited group is to be compared, depending on which comparison group is used. The rate of advanced breast cancer in the population of women aged 50–69 in East Anglia remained fairly stable over the 10-year period 1976–86. However, there was a sudden marked increase in the two years 1987–88 immediately preceding the introduction of screening (McCann *et al.*, 1998). This led to difficulty in estimating the screening-induced reduction in advanced cancer since the rate of advanced cancer expected in the absence of screening varies depending on the method of prediction used. In the figure, three methods have been used to predict the incidence of stage II–IV cancers expected in 1997 in the absence of screening. Method 1: the rate of advanced cancers observed in previous years (1976–86 in Method 1a, or 1976–88 in Method 1b) has been projected forward to 1997 assuming that trends in incidence observed in the previous years will continue to 1997 at a constant rate. Method 2: the rate in 1997 is estimated as the average rate seen over the period 1987–88. Method 3: the ratio of advanced to early cancers seen during the period 1989–96 in women who had not yet received an invitation to screening was applied to the total number of cases actually observed in 1997 to generate an expected advanced cancer rate.

8.4 Sources of data

Having established the information requirements for breast screening programme evaluation,

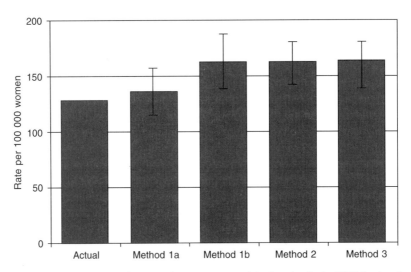

Figure 8.1 Predicting the rate of advanced cancer expected in East Anglia in 1997 in the absence of screening. Method 1: the rate of advanced cancers observed in previous years (1976–86 in Method 1a, or 1976–88 in Method 1b) has been projected forward to 1997 assuming a constant rate of change. Method 2: assumes the rate in 1997 will be the same as the average rate seen over the period 1987–88. Method 3: the ratio of advanced to early cancers seen during the period 1989–96 in women who had not yet received an invitation to screening was applied to the total number of cases actually observed in 1997 to generate an expected advanced cancer rate

the sources and methods required for data acquisition must be considered. In the UK, population-based information on cancer incidence is available from regional Cancer Registries. However, the availability and quality of the data vary considerably between registries. Since 1960, East Anglia has benefited from a high-quality cancer registration system. Using information from pathology laboratories, clinical records and death certificates (and, to a lesser extent, from GPs, post-mortem examinations and private clinics), the Cancer Registry records every case of cancer that affects residents in the region and follows the case until death. The Registry has a high reputation, both nationally and internationally, for the completeness, timeliness and validity of its data. It is one of the few registries in the UK that has, from the beginning, collected data on breast cancer stage at diagnosis (with the majority of the cases being staged by a clinical oncologist) and performed active follow-up of patients (de Bono and Kingsley Pillers, 1978). Cases are followed up three years after diagnosis, and again every five years until death; thus vital status information is reliable and up to date. Since the start of the screening programme, the Registry has operated a policy of 'fast tracking' all breast cancer registrations, ensuring rapidity of case registration and enabling more meaningful and timely evaluation. For areas where cancer registration does not include such clinical details as stage, other information sources will be required, including treatment centres and pathology laboratories.

The Cancer Registry therefore provides information on all breast cancer cases occurring in the target population for the screening programme. It is noteworthy here that, since a screening programme is likely to have an upper age limit as well as a lower one, the age range to be monitored requires careful thought. The rate of interval cancers is of crucial importance in screening programme evaluation (Day *et al.*, 1995), and one needs to follow up the oldest invited age group for an agreed length of time after their final screen to ascertain whether or not they remain disease-free. In East Anglia, we want to follow up the 64-year-olds for an additional three years (i.e. until their 68th birthdays) for accurate interval cancer monitoring. It is also worth noting incidentally, that as screening prevents not immediate but future mortality, some of the future mortality benefit will accrue to women after they have passed the upper age limit for screening. In fact, because of the ready availability of population statistics by five-year age band, and the common epidemiological practice of analysing rates by these five-year age bands, it is convenient to use the four age groups 50–54, 55–59, 60–64 and 65–69 years as the target age groups for monitoring.

Collection of information from the Cancer Registry on all cases in the population in the age range of interest should be on a regular basis, by computer download of the relevant information. This information may then require manual supplementation with additional information obtained from cancer registration cards, clinical notes and pathology reports. The data from the East Anglia Cancer Registry on all cases in the target age range for the evaluation of the screening programme in East Anglia includes personal information (name, date of birth, address, etc.) as well as clinical and pathological details of cases (date of diagnosis, stage, malignancy grade, lesion size, node status, etc.).

It is essential that a clear set of definitions is drawn up at the outset of the evaluation and rigorously adhered to throughout the entire study period. This will ensure data consistency throughout the study duration despite the long period of time over which data are to be collected, and the inevitable changes in data collection and registry staff, registry policy, and even international definitions (e.g. changes in UICC staging criteria (UICC 1978, 1987, 1997)). Wherever possible, a copy of the original pathology report for all cases should be obtained, reviewed and stored. These should be used in conjunction with registry data whose pathology details can be cross-checked or augmented with those on the report. Discrepancies can be addressed with registry staff so that any differences of opinion are resolved; thus the exercise can provide a useful quality control mechanism in the registration process. Clear rules on data classification and coding must be established. These include which system of malignancy grading should be used, and how grade information from different systems can be interpreted and coded; how lesions will be staged if lymph nodes are not sampled; and how many nodes should be sampled and found to be disease-free before the case can be classified as node negative. The complete dataset should be collected from the start of the programme and, if the historical cohort approach is to be adopted, for a sufficient number of years before the start of screening to give reliable baseline information on the pre-screening burden of the disease. This length of time will depend on magnitude and temporal variability of incidence rates (McCann *et al.*, 1998, and Figure 8.1).

8.5 Categorisation of cases according to detection mode

Having described the cancer baseline in the absence of screening, the next step is to allocate cases arising after the introduction of screening into groups according to their mode of detection. Such allocation allows further analysis of the effects of screening by comparison of differences in stage and other prognostic indicators in the invited and comparison group.

Attention must be paid, however, to the effect of length bias, as described above. Length bias is the tendency for screening to detect a disproportionate number of cancers which spend a long time in the preclinical detectable phase (PCDP) which is the time during which cancers are detectable by screening but not yet clinically evident. A long duration of PCDP suggests that these cancers are relatively slow growing and thus have a good prognosis. The effect of length bias is mainly concentrated in the prevalence screen, since tumours with a very long PCDP tend to need only one screen to detect them. To remove the effect of length bias, all cancers arising in a period running from immediately after the first screen to immediately after the second screen are grouped together and compared with the uninvited group. This set of cancers has been termed the unbiased set (Duffy *et al.*, 1991). Thus the unbiased set comprises the cancers arising as intervals after the first screen, plus cancers arising in women who were invited but did not attend the first screen, plus those detected at the second screen. Note that, in this method, the non-attenders have been included with the screened women since we are comparing cancers arising in the entire *invited* population with those arising over a similar time period in our comparison group.

The following categories of detection mode for all cancers occurring in women within the target age range are suggested:

- *Screen detected*. These are cancers detected as a result of a positive screen.
- *Interval cancer*. Cancers that occur in women screened negative before the next screen is due.
- *Non-attender*. These are cancers arising in women who were invited but never attended for screening. This group will usually include those whom the programme failed to contact due, for example, to moving house, as well as those who decided not to attend. One might wish to identify such individuals as a separate category.
- *Lapsed attender*. These are cancers arising in women who have attended for screening but who develop cancer having failed to attend subsequent invitations. We would include here women who have attended but who are now over the age range for invitation and do not self-refer for screening. It might be desirable to distinguish these women from women who received further invitation(s) but declined to attend. Note that we distinguish this group from the above non-attender group who have never attended for screening.
- *Pre-invitation*. Cancers arising in women before they receive an invitation for screening.
- *Outside age range*. Cancers arising in women who were above the upper age limit for invitation, but still within the study age range, at the time screening was introduced in their area of residence (i.e. between the ages of 65 and 69, in our study).
- *Never invited*. Cancers in women who have never received an invitation for screening.

Classification of cases into these categories requires knowledge of their screening invitation history. For the breast screening programme, this information is available from the screening centres. In East Anglia we collect information on invitation histories for all women invited for screening by regular computer download. As with cases registered by the Cancer Registry, personal details of all women invited for screening are collected (name, address and date of birth), together with information on all screening invitations (including dates and outcomes) and, for screen-detected breast cancers, the diagnosis date and pathology details (lesion size, malignancy grade, invasive status, node status and histological subtype).

By computer matching of registered cancer cases and women invited for screening, it is possible to allocate the majority of registered cases into one of the seven categories of detection mode. The matching program used in East Anglia is a custom written program based on *Soundex* (Knuth, 1973) which matches on surname, forename and date of birth. In our program, various levels of stringency of matching can be selected, for example using only part of the name and date/month/year of birth in order to determine the likelihood of successful matching. We check all matches manually for concordance of address details between the two data sources. An initial round of stringent matching is run to link the majority of cases then, for cases which do not match, a less stringent 'trawl' is performed. A policy must be adopted for dealing with non-matching cases, which should be rare. In East Anglia we have recruited the help of the Health Authorities who hold the details of all patients registered with GPs and from whom the screening centres obtain population lists of women for invitation for screening. Staff at the Health Authorities have been invaluable in tracing women who have moved or changed their names or whose date of birth or address details require verification.

If case matching is a tedious process, allocation into categories of detection mode is more arduous still. For each match, categorisation is determined by examining the screening invitation dates and outcomes for the presence or absence of invitation, attendance or non-attendance at screening, and for diagnosis or no diagnosis of cancer at screening. By comparing this information with the diagnosis date recorded at the Cancer Registry, all cancer cases may be categorised into one of the categories described above (Patnick and Muir Gray, 1993; McCann *et al.*, 1998). In East Anglia this is done manually. Positive matches should be stored as a database, possibly using the Cancer Registry download as a 'backbone' and adding in extra fields, depending on the file structure of Cancer Registry and screening unit downloaded files.

The screening information we store in East Anglia includes the identifying code of the screening centre who issued the invitation, the date of the relevant invitation or screen, the relevant screen number (first screen, second, third, etc.) and also invitation number (in case, e.g. women failed to attend the original invitation but attended on the second invitation), the referral code for the relevant screening appointment (first screen, routine rescreen, self-referral, early rescreen) and finally the outcome of the screening appointment (not attended, cancer detected, screen normal, normal following assessment, early recall, etc.).

8.6 Issues to be considered when categorising cancers

Case matching for screen detected cancers is usually straightforward because the screening centre will in principle have details of all these. The non-attenders are less straightforward, not least because a considerable proportion of them may have failed to attend because they were already undergoing investigation for a breast abnormality or because they were on follow-up from a previous breast cancer. In East Anglia, there is a policy of checking on any case which is diagnosed within six months of an unattended screening invitation. With the help of the screening centres' breast care nurses, we examine the hospital notes to determine the initial date of medical contact concerning the abnormality (this is usually the date the woman first consulted her general practitioner regarding a breast symptom). This date is used to decide whether or not a case should be categorised as a 'non-attender'. If the date the patient first sought medical help regarding the abnormality precedes the date of invitation then, in East Anglia, we would categorise this case as 'pre-invitation' despite the fact that the date of diagnosis recorded at the Cancer Registry was after the date of the unattended screening appointment.

A further complication sometimes encountered in population screening programmes relates to the protocol of data storage on the screening unit computer system. The computer system designed for a screening programme is often appointment-based, rather than person-based. As a consequence of this, if a woman gives advance notice of her intention not to attend a particular appointment offered, this appointment will be reallocated to someone else and the invitation data will be lost from the original invitee's records. This poses significant problems in the evaluation process and in some cases in East Anglia we have resorted to re-creating appointments based on dates of birth, areas of residence, and screening invitation schedules. Once again, the Health Authorities have been of assistance since they keep a fuller record of each woman's complete invitation history, albeit with fewer outcome details. Staff at the Health Authorities have been most helpful in searching records to help re-create screening histories for women who are apparently missing appointments. This exercise has brought to light interesting data on movement in and out of the region, and on the numbers of women whose names have been removed at the request of their general practitioners before the screening units sent out the invitations.

The interval cancer group has its own complications. At the outset, one needs to consider how one is defining an interval cancer. An interval cancer is a cancer arising in a woman screened negative before the next screen is due. When is the next screen due? The obvious answer is after a time equal to the inter-screen interval. However, although there will be a policy laid down by the screening programme which defines how often women should be screened, screening centres may not strictly adhere to this and there may be early rescreening or, alternatively, 'slippage' (Faux et al., 1997).

Early rescreening is only partially addressed by using 'woman years at risk' as the denominator (Breslow and Day, 1987) when calculating interval cancer rates as opposed to the more straightforward 'number of women screened negative'. This is because interval cancer rates increase with time after negative screen and, if the next screen is early, the risk per unit time of an interval cancer will be less than if the agreed inter-screen interval were used, thus will not give a true indication of the effectiveness of the agreed screening cycle. A mathematical adjustment of interval cancer rates may be made to allow for this if required (Day et al., 1995).

Slippage, on the other hand, is the case where due to resource-related or organisational problems the actual invitation to the next screen occurs later than scheduled. This will mean that some cancers may present symptomatically in women after the agreed inter-screen interval has elapsed, and following the previous (negative) screen but before the actual date of reinvitation. In this situation, if the target inter-screen interval is used as a cut off, the case will not be counted (indeed, it does not fit into any category). Interval cancer rates will then not be a true representation of that screening centre's performance and the weakness in the centre's performance will pass unobserved. For this reason, one might consider using the mean inter-screen interval for each screening centre as the cut-off time for follow up. However, this mean inter-screen interval may vary significantly between screening centres and this may cause problems depending on the nature of the research question being addressed. Comparability with national targets and with other programmes may also be relevant issues, in addition to comparison of individual screening centres' performance. It is thus advisable to enter the data, including all cancers, using as flexible a coding as possible so that data can easily be reclassified in order best to address the issue in question. Storage of invitation dates as well as diagnosis dates allows calculation of the inter-screen interval. A combination of the required inter-screen interval plus detection mode classification as 'interval cancer' can be used to select only those cases of current interest, and the rest can be reclassified as appropriate. It is definitely advisable to retain information on all cancers and to ascertain as exactly as possible the time since last negative screen in all cases.

The effect of variation in follow-up time for identifying interval cancers on number of cases, woman years and interval cancer rates is shown for the East Anglian prevalence round in Table 8.1. The screening interval in the UK programme should be three years. However, in reality there is variation between screening units in the actual time to reinvitation, and some slippage. In this table, we show interval cancers, women years (wy) at risk and incidence rates of interval cancers. Data are shown for the interval following the East Anglian programme's prevalence screen, and using four different default follow-up times for those women with no scheduled reinvitation: the mean time between appointments for each screening unit: $2\frac{1}{2}$ years; 3 years; and $3\frac{1}{2}$ years. Note that use of different default follow-up times affects both the absolute numbers of cases and woman years and the interval cancer incidence rates per 10 000 woman years. This effect is most marked for the oldest age group for whom a default time had to be used frequently, since this group did not usually have a scheduled rescreen. It is worth noting, however, that the variation can be by as much as 10% in the age group 55–59.

In addition to identifying interval cancers through computer matching with the Cancer Registry, further cases may be notified by the screening centres themselves. This can be used as a fail-safe approach to ensure that case ascertainment is as high as possible.

It must be stressed how important it is to be exhaustive in the search for interval cancers because, unless all the cases are identified, any evaluation based on interval cancer rates will be incorrect and misleading. Poor-quality cancer registration or identification of interval cases will lead to underestimation of interval cancer rates and hence overestimation of programme performance. Excellent cancer registration and exhaustive record linkage are therefore essential in the evaluation process.

The importance of correctly ascertaining true rates for interval cancers is illustrated in Table 8.2 which shows how the predicted mortality reduction which could be achieved by a screening programme varies directly with interval cancer rates. Three-year interval cancer rates have been used to predict the likely reduction in mortality that a screening programme may achieve (see Day et al., 1995, for the method). These are expressed as a combined proportionate incidence, i.e. as the proportion of incident cancers arising as interval cancers in the inter-screening period. The proportionate incidence (PI) of interval cancers in a given year ($i = 1, 2, 3$) after a negative screen is defined as:

$$\text{PI}(\text{year } i) = \frac{\text{interval cancer rate in year } i}{\text{underlying incidence in year } i}$$

where the underlying incidence is the expected incidence of breast cancer in the absence of screening. For a three-year inter-screening period, the combined proportionate incidence of interval cancers is

$$\tfrac{1}{3}[\text{PI}(\text{year } 1) + \text{PI}(\text{year } 2) + \text{PI}(\text{year } 3)]$$

Table 8.1 Effect of follow-up period on age-specific interval cancer rates

	Period of follow-up											
	Mean inter-screen interval			$2\frac{1}{2}$ years			3 years			$3\frac{1}{2}$ years		
Age group at diagnosis	Cases	Woman years	Rate per 10^4 wy	Cases	Woman years	Rate per 10^4 wy	Cases	Woman years	Rate per 10^4 wy	Cases	Woman years	Rate per 10^4 wy
50–54	112	105 895	10.58	97	95 065	10.20	113	104 913	10.77	113	106 468	10.61
55–59	152	146 645	10.37	117	121 010	9.67	152	144 848	10.49	158	148 855	10.61
60–64	153	131 901	11.60	119	110 079	10.81	150	130 302	11.51	157	134 636	11.66
65–69	39	34 566	11.28	21	23 599	8.90	37	33 710	10.98	51	44 661	11.42
50–69	**456**	**419 007**	**10.88**	**354**	**349 753**	**10.12**	**452**	**413 773**	**10.92**	**479**	**434 620**	**11.02**

Table 8.2 Effect of interval cancer incidence on expected reduction in breast cancer mortality, women aged 50–64

Interval cancers (Combined proportionate incidence)	Breast cancer mortality reduction (%) in:		
	Screened women (100% compliance)	Total population (70% compliance)	Total population (80% compliance)
34%	39	24	29
40%	35	22	26
50%	29	19	22
54%	27	18	21
60%	24	15	18
66%	20	13	15

Figures in the table are based on the expected fatality from screen-detected cancers, interval cancers and cancers in non-attenders, estimated from the results of the Swedish Two-County Trial of breast cancer screening (Tabar *et al.*, 1985). Note how the predicted mortality reduction varies with interval cancer proportionate incidence, particularly when compliance is high.

A more fundamental problem in categorisation of cancers is that different organisations (e.g. Cancer Registry and screening centres) may use different definitions of cancer. In East Anglia, the Cancer Registry only registers primary cancers. Strict rules are applied in deciding whether a lesion constitutes a new primary or a recurrence (UICC, 1978, 1987, 1997; Ainsworth *et al.*, 1993). Bilateral cancers and ipsilateral simultaneous multiple primaries further complicate the issue. In the UK, there is the anomaly that, although the breast screening programme counts as a cancer any lesion detected in the breast by screening, be it a new primary or a recurrence, it only scores the woman once. The East Anglian Cancer Registry, on the other hand, scores cancers not women, but will not register recurrences nor score as breast malignancy any lesion in the breast other than ICD-10 C50 or D05 (Ainsworth *et al.*, 1993; WHO, 1992). Further problems arise in the handling of microinvasion, which the breast screening programme includes with non-invasive cancers but which, if definitely present, the Cancer Registry counts as invasive cancer. These issues may sound trivial but do require rigorous and consistent handling. Using strict Cancer Registry guidelines is usually the best option because, for categories of cancer other than screen-detected and interval, only Cancer Registry data will be available. Furthermore, if the comparison group (the 'baseline') has been identified from Cancer Registry records, then Cancer Registry rules will have been used to define this group and comparison with a differently defined group would not be valid. However, screening units may be dissatisfied with figures in which not every woman who has a lesion detected is scored. Further problems with this approach may arise if interval cancer or screen-detected cancer data are being compared with other regions/programmes where different classification rules have been applied. It is important to seek agreement among all parties involved in the evaluation from the outset.

8.7 Conclusions

Evaluation of a screening programme is not for the faint-hearted. It must be approached with rigour, an obsession for detail, and a clearly defined protocol for all stages of the process. Analysis will require collection of large amounts of data on both the study population and an appropriately chosen comparison group. All data sources must be verified for accuracy and completeness since errors, for example in data coding, are found in the unlikeliest of places. Sources of bias and inaccuracy are everywhere. The rewards of a robust evaluation are, however, either the reassurance that the screening programme is on target to achieve the full possible benefit in disease morbidity and mortality or the facts with which to identify areas where change is needed and with which to persuade screening staff to improve performance.

References

Ainsworth, A., Gravestock, S., Linklater, L. and Page, M. (1993). *Information and Training Manual for Cancer Registration in England and Wales*. UKACR, London.

Breslow, N.E. and Day, N.E. (1987). *Statistical Methods in Cancer Research II. The Design and Analysis of Cohort Studies*. International Agency for Research on Cancer, Lyon, pp. 48–79.

Day, N.E. (1996). The theoretical basis for cancer screening. In Miller, A.B. (ed.), *Advances in Cancer Screening*. Kluwer Academic Publishers, Boston, pp. 9–24.

Day, N.E., Williams, D.R.R. and Khaw, K.T. (1989). Breast cancer screening programmes: the development of a monitoring and evaluation system. *Br. J. Cancer*, **59**, 954–8.

Day, N.E., McCann, J., Camilleri-Ferrante, C.C., Britton, P., Hurst, G., Cush, S. and Duffy, S. (1995). Monitoring interval cancers in breast screening programmes: the East Anglian experience. *J. Med. Screening*, **2**, 180–5.

De Bono, A.M. and Kingsley Pillers, E.M. (1978). Carcinoma of the breast in East Anglia 1960–1975: a changing pattern of presentation? *J. Epidemiol. Comm. Health*, **32**, 178–82.

Duffy, S.W., Tabar, L., Fagerberg, G. *et al.* (1991). Breast screening, prognostic factors and survival: results from the Swedish two-county study. *Br. J. Cancer*, **64**, 1133–8.

Faux, A.M., Richardson, D.C., Lawrence, G.M., Wheaton, M.E. and Wallis, M.G. (1997). Interval breast cancers in the NHS Breast Screening Programme: does the current definition exclude too many? *J. Med. Screening*, **4**, 169–73.

Forrest, P. (1986). *Breast Cancer Screening*. HMSO, London.

Hennekens, C.H. and Buring, J.E. (1987). Evaluation of screening programmes: feasibility and efficacy. In: Mayrent, S.L. (ed.), *Epidemiology in Medicine*. Little, Brown and Co., Boston, pp. 335–47.

Knuth, D.E. (1973). *The Art of Computer Programming, Sorting and Searching*. **3**, Addison-Wesley Wokingham, pp. 389–402.

McCann, J., Stockton, D. and Day, N.E. (1998). Breast cancer in East Anglia: the impact of the breast screening programme on stage at diagnosis. *J. Med. Screening*, **5**, 42–8.

Patnick, J. and Muir Gray, J.A. (1993). Guidelines on the collection and use of breast cancer data. *NHS Breast Screening Programme Publication No. 26*. HMSO, London.

Tabar, L., Gad, A., Holmberg, L.H. *et al.* (1985). Reduction in breast cancer mortality by mass screening with mammography: first results of a randomised trial in two Swedish counties. *Lancet*, **I**, 829–32.

Tabar, L., Fagerberg, C.J.G., Day, N.E. and Holmberg, L. (1987). The Swedish two-county breast cancer screening trial: update and initial results on the screening interval. *Br. J. Cancer*, **55**, 547–51.

UICC (1978, 1987, 1997). *TNM Classification of Malignant Tumours*, 3rd, 4th. 5th Edn. Springer-Verlag, New York.

WHO (1992). ICD-10: *International Statistical Classification of Diseases and Related Health Problems*. 10th Revision. World Health Organisation, Geneva.

9

Use of routine data to monitor and evaluate cervical screening

Peter D. Sasieni

9.1 Introduction

Population screening as a means of disease prevention has become increasingly common since the 1960s. The English National Cervical Screening Programme aims to screen women aged 20–64 at least once every five years. The financial cost of such a programme is huge and yet cervical screening has never been demonstrated, by means of a randomised controlled clinical trial, to reduce the incidence of or mortality from cervical cancer. Today the vast majority of experts believe that cytological screening does prevent invasive cervical cancer and that a randomised trial of cytological screening versus no screening would be unethical. Many questions, however, remain unanswered. For instance:

- What precisely is the magnitude of protection from cervical screening?
- What is the benefit of screening every 2, 3, 4 or 5 years?
- Up to what age should women who have had several negative tests continue to be screened?

It is possible that ethically acceptable studies could be designed to address certain questions, but the cost and time required to obtain definitive answers makes such studies unlikely ever to be conducted. Indeed, by the time a 15-year study is completed, the current cytological test may well have been replaced by some new or modified procedure. Alternatively, one could try to estimate the effectiveness of screening by analysing individuals within a population that is subject to screening. A possible approach, which has been frequently adopted for cervical screening evaluation, is the case-control design.

Cervical screening is designed to prevent invasive cancer by detecting and treating lesions at a preinvasive or even a premalignant phase, but may also lead to early detection of cancer. This should be contrasted to mammography, which saves lives through detection of occult breast tumours, but does not detect precancerous conditions and cannot, therefore, reduce the incidence of cancer.

9.2 Natural history

Before considering different study designs in greater detail, we first review the natural history of cervical cancer. There is little information from studies that directly observe the development of cervical cancer because it is generally felt to be unethical not to treat precancerous cervical disease. Most of our knowledge is derived from the follow-up of women with smear test abnormalities and the study of the incidence and prevalence of cervical lesions.

Cervical neoplasia appears to constitute a continuum ranging from cervical intraepithelial neoplasia (CIN) grades I to III, to microinvasive and fully invasive cancer. The vast majority of cervical cancers have certain types of the human papillomavirus (HPV) DNA within the tumour. It is estimated that at least 90% of cervical cancer is caused by these HPVs (Bosch *et al.*, 1995). CIN I is frequently not associated with HPV infection and may not therefore be part of the continuum (Kiviat *et al.*, 1992). However, histology is not able to distinguish between CIN I associated with an oncogenic HPV infection and CIN I without HPV DNA. The histological report of HPV is based on morphological features and is not particularly tightly correlated with the presence of oncogenic HPV DNA (Korobowicz *et al.*, 1997).

Longitudinal studies on young women show that the majority of HPV infections are transient (Hildesheim *et al.*, 1994; Wheeler *et al.*, 1996) and that the virus is sexually transmitted (Burk *et al.*, 1996; Dillner *et al.*, 1996). Persistence of the infection has been shown to be associated with the development of cervical lesions (Koutsky *et al.,* 1992; Remmink *et al.*, 1995; Ho *et al.*, 1995) and viral load can be used as a surrogate for persistence (Cuzick, 1997; Brisson *et al.*, 1996). It is widely assumed that integration of the viral DNA into the host genome is one of the key steps in the development of cancer (Cullen *et al.*, 1991), although some carcinomas only have episomal viral DNA (Das *et al.*, 1992). The vast majority of HPV infections do not lead to cancer, but are dealt with by the host's immune system.

Figure 9.1 illustrates the natural history of cervical neoplasia. Percentages on the arrows are approximate lifetime progression or regression probabilities. A percentage within a box represents the approximate lifetime risk of reaching that state assuming no screening and no treatment of cervical cancer. The diagram is a simplification showing only the main routes of progression and regression. It does not, for instance, allow for a small proportion of high-grade disease developing without prior HPV infection, nor does it show that progression following a persistent HPV infection is far more likely than after a newly incident or transient infection. Follow-up studies of women with CIN have found that about 60% of CIN I regresses compared to about 33% of CIN III; 11% and 22% of CIN I and II, respectively, progressed to CIN III (Ostor, 1993). Other groups claim rather greater progression rates. For instance Campion *et al.* (1986) found that 26% of lesions cytologically and colposcopically consistent with CIN I progressed to histologically proven CIN III. It has been estimated that the mean duration of CIN is about 12 years and that the time from HPV infection to CIN is typically between 1 and 10 years (van Ballegooijen *et al.*, 1997). Approximately one-third of CIN III are expected to progress to cervical cancer, if left untreated, over a period of 15 years. However, there is still considerable uncertainty as to progression and regression estimates.

Figure 9.2 shows CIN III rates by age. Rates for England and Wales are for registrations of carcinoma *in situ* per 100 000 women in 1992 (Office of National Statistics, 1998).

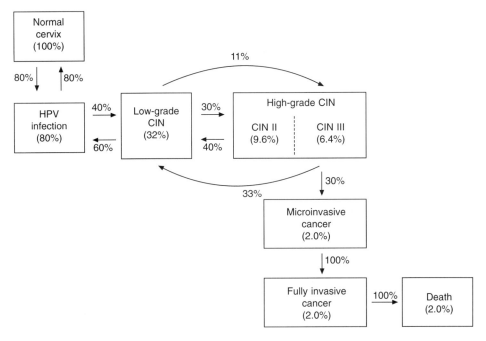

Figure 9.1 Natural history of cervical neoplasia

Rates for south-west Hampshire are adjusted for screening coverage: they are per 100 000 women screened in the preceding 3.5 years (Herbert and Smith, 1999). Note that whereas the figures for England and Wales underestimate the true rate of disease (differentially in those under age 20 and over age 50), the adjustment to the

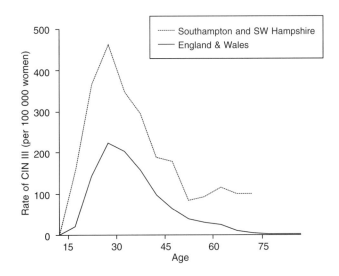

Figure 9.2 CIN III rates as a function of age, England and Wales and south-west Hampshire

data from south-west Hampshire will tend to exaggerate the disease incidence, particularly in those age groups in which only women at high risk have cervical smears.

CIN III is very rare in women under the age of 20. The rates rise rapidly, peaking at about age 30, and fall again more slowly, being at about half their peak by age 40 and just 10–20% of their maximum by age 50 (Evans *et al.*, 1997). These rates are probably a mixture of incidence and prevalence and are also affected by the increasing incidence of cervical disease in younger women in several Western countries, most notably England and Wales.

9.3 Cohort data

It is useful to consider what one might do given data on a large cohort of women before attempting to resolve the design and analysis issues in less ambitious studies. In an ideal situation we might have a randomised study of three- versus five-yearly screening. Comparison of the risks of dying from cervical cancer between the two arms is straightforward. We are also interested in the extent to which more frequent screening prevents incidence of cervical cancer. Having demonstrated a difference in mortality, we could compare the cancer incidence rates in the two arms with the knowledge that if no difference is found then the reduction in mortality probably resulted from early detection and successful treatment of cancer. Analysis of stage-specific incidence might demonstrate a significant reduction in late-stage cancers with no difference or even an increase in early cancers. Since the five-year survival rate of stage I cancer is around 80%, but that of stage IV is only around 10% (Miller *et al.*, 1993), such a shift in stage would be of great importance.

The identification of screen-detected tumours is important in breast screening, which reduces mortality through early detection of cancer, but seems less helpful in cervical screening. Ideally cervical screening will identify precancerous lesions so, other than in the first round of screening, the proportion of screen-detected cases should be small. An increase in the proportion of screen-detected tumours will only be beneficial if early detection leads to prolonged survival. Demonstrating the latter is complicated by lead-time and length bias (see Chapter 1).

In the absence of a randomised trial one must analyse the data by the observed screening history rather than some predetermined random allocation. Inevitably one will be unable to control for selection bias if women at highest risk of developing cervical cancer are more likely to opt out of screening. However, the possibility of this being a serious problem will be small if the association with screening remains after adjusting for known risk factors such as number of sexual partners.

Ignoring the problem of selection bias, how should one classify screening histories? In analogy with the hypothetical randomised trial we would like some measure of a woman's usual screening interval if such a thing exists. A non-negative screening test leads to suspension of the routine recall and to more frequent repeat tests. Thus, the relationship between the outcome variable (cancer incidence) and the exposure variable (dates and results of screening tests) is complicated. Bearing in mind that a non-negative smear or diagnosis of a precancerous lesion will alter the course of future screening, one may choose to classify women based on their screening history up to their first non-negative smear. Figure 9.3 illustrates the complications of attempting to characterise a woman's

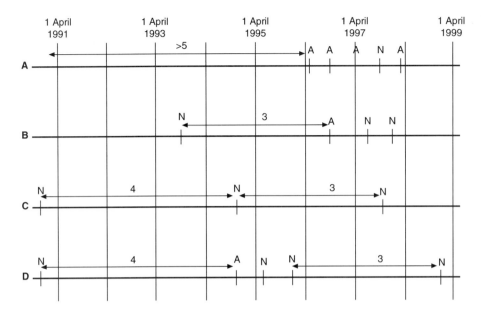

Figure 9.3 Schematic diagram of four screening histories, showing times of negative (N) and abnormal (A) smears

screening interval using this method, in the context of a programme whose usual recall interval changed from four years to three in 1995. Four hypothetical screening histories are shown:

Woman A: This woman has had five smears since April 1996, but since the first of these was abnormal her 'usual' screening interval is defined by the period before this first abnormal screen. It is at least five years.

Woman B: This woman had an abnormal smear in October 1996, having had a normal smear three years earlier, so her interval is three years.

Woman C: This woman has never had an abnormal smear and, since the change to the programme, her screening interval is three years.

Woman D: Although this woman's most recent interval was three years, it was preceded by a non-negative smear. Her interval is therefore four years, the time from the last negative smear to the first non-negative.

There are two disadvantages of such an approach. The first may arise if there have been temporal changes to the screening programme. Suppose, for instance, that over the past four years the most common screening interval has been reduced from four to three yearly. Then a woman who had an abnormal smear four years ago would on average have a longer screening interval (prior to abnormality) than one who had never had a non-negative result. This is illustrated by woman C and woman D in Figure 9.3. An attraction of the case-control approach (see Section 9.4) is that such a woman could be matched to others whose screening histories would also be classified based only on events prior to the date of the abnormal result of the first woman.

The other weakness of considering screening only up to a woman's first non-negative test is that it says nothing about the subsequent management of that woman. Since approximately 5% of routine cervical smears are non-negative, a population repeatedly screened will contain a substantial number of women who have had a non-negative result. A full evaluation of a screening programme should include an analysis of subsequent screening and treatment for this important subgroup.

In analysis of a non-randomised cohort study, one would attempt to estimate the same effects as in a randomised trial, albeit with perhaps greater analytic difficulty and more caution in interpretation. For example, based on the best arbitration of a woman's typical interval, one would wish to compare incidence rates of invasive cervical cancer, and stage of disease, between intervals. One might even wish to compare mortality from cervical cancer. It should be borne in mind, however, that a cohort subject to effective screening would have to be very large to confer sufficient power for internal comparison of mortality, and even of invasive cancer incidence. For this reason, much of the past work on cervical cancer screening evaluation has used the case-control design.

9.4 Case-control studies using morbidity

The case-control study has the advantage of using considerably fewer resources per disease case than a cohort study. This is especially true for invasive cervical cancer in a screened population, since if the screening is effective, the disease will be very rare. It is also flexible and can be designed specifically for investigation of individual issues. It is, however, prone to various biases and has the same problems of classification of screening histories as are encountered in a cohort study. In particular, it is problematic defining a woman's screening interval when a non-negative finding at a given screen shortens the interval to the next. It also requires caution in interpretation in the presence of both screen-detected and symptomatic cancers, since the purpose of the screening is to prevent the cancer from occurring. The classical solution, adopted by a large international study of cervical screening (IARC, 1986), addresses these two problems. It distinguishes between screen-detected and other cancers and analyses the time from the most recent negative smear. Controls for non-screen-detected cancers are chosen at random (matched on age) from the population, whereas controls for screen-detected cases are chosen conditionally on having had a smear test taken at about the same time as the case. This design was adopted to match away the bias that might otherwise arise from the fact that a screen-detected case must have participated in the screening programme and the time to her previous negative test will be her most recent screening interval. However, by insisting that the control for a screen detected case has had a test within a given six-month period, one is more likely to select a control who is screened very frequently, and that introduces a bias. Defining exposure as the time from a previous negative smear is not completely satisfactory either. It addresses the question of whether screening can detect a precancerous lesion, but not whether there is any benefit to the woman of having such a lesion detected. In other words, the relative protection associated with screening estimated from analysis of the time to the previous negative result will only be achieved in a population if a woman with a positive test result will never go on to develop invasive cancer.

First we briefly consider the question of who should be a case. One possibility is to consider women who have died of cancer. An advantage of such a definition is that screening has clearly failed. There are however several disadvantages stemming from the time from cancer incidence to death. Since screening can only intervene before cancer diagnosis, studying cancer deaths requires considering screening several years further back and reliable data may not be available. Even when information is reliable, it will reflect on screening as it was several years ago, not on the current situation. Further, cytological screening is intended to reduce the incidence of cervical cancer. For these reasons it is important to include all women with primary invasive cervical cancers as cases. It will be useful to distinguish three kinds of case: (1) screen-detected, (2) symptomatic and (3) post-mortem. Cervical cancers diagnosed only post-mortem are rare and could be regarded for practical purposes as a subset of the symptomatic cases, so we do not consider them further here.

We now consider a variety of approaches to selection of controls and the subsequent analysis of case-control data for cervical cancer. Cases and controls should be selected from the same defined population so that each case would have been eligible as a control had she not developed cancer and conversely each control would have been included as a case had she developed cancer. All controls should be at risk of cervical cancer at the time of diagnosis of the case. Thus matching by age, and possibly by other temporal factors, is necessary. In particular, women who have had a hysterectomy no longer have a cervix and should not, therefore, be eligible as a control for a case with cancer diagnosed after the date of the hysterectomy. Controls should be matched, as far as possible, for access to screening. This is very difficult to define, but surrogates such as neighbourhood, general practitioner or address-based socioeconomic status should be considered.

9.4.1 Random (age-matched) controls

The simplest approach to selection of controls is to use random age-matched women from the population register. Such controls are suitable for asymptomatic cases, but are not directly comparable with screen-detected cases. The latter must have been screened at least once and, excluding the smear that led to the diagnosis of cancer, the time to their last (previous) smear will be equal to their usual screening interval. By contrast, the controls need never have been screened and the time since an individual's last smear will, on average, be half the length of her usual screening interval. It is possible, however, using the technical statistical principles of renewal theory (Cox, 1962), to quantify the expected difference between the distribution of time since last smear between screen-detected cases and random controls, and therefore to adjust for it in analysis. This assumes that we are only counting routine smears, since the interval between 'repeats following a previous abnormal' will have a different (shorter) distribution. Thus it is possible in principle to compare screen-detected cases to randomly selected controls *provided* one is aware of the problem of repeat versus routine smears.

9.4.2 Screened controls

This method is discussed because it has become the standard approach, but it is not satisfactory because, as we have mentioned, the controls will over-represent women who are screened more frequently. The idea is to select a control for a screen-detected case from women who were screened at the same time (in practice within a few months) as the diagnostic smear of the case. The following extreme example illustrates the magnitude of the bias that could result from naive use of such controls. Suppose that:

1. one-fifth of the population goes to each of 1, 2, 3, 4, 5-yearly screening,
2. half of all cancers have no occult phase and half have an occult phase that lasts more than 5 years, and
3. there is no beneficial effect of screening (but it will discover cancers during the occult phase).

Odds ratios for screen-detected cancer relative to the screened controls are calculated according to the time since last smear. Although there is no benefit from screening, the expected value of the odds ratio for women last screened over four years before inclusion in the study relative to those screened within the past year is 5.0. This follows simply because one expects five times as many new occult cancers to have developed in those who have not been screened for five years than in those who were screened just a year ago.

9.4.3 Weighted screened controls

Here we propose a method of weighting which involves estimating the renewal intensity. Define the case's index smear as the smear that eventually leads to the diagnosis. Consider a one-year interval $I = (T - 1, T]$ containing the case's index smear.

1. Select at random a control with a screening test in I.
2. Look at all routine smears in the previous six years $(T - 6, T]$. Let T_0 denote the time of the index smear and $T_{-1}, ..., T_{-r}$ the times of the other r routine smears in the interval.
3. Define $\mu_1 = (T_0 - T_{-r})/r$ if $r > 0$ and $\mu_1 = 7$ if $r = 0$. Let $\mu_2 = 6.5/(r + 1)$. Then estimate the smear intensity by the average time between smears $\mu = \max(\mu_1, \mu_2)$ and use the control with weight $w = 1/\mu = \min(1/\mu_1, 1/\mu_2)$.

The idea here is simply to weight the controls to take into account the fact that women who are screened more often are more likely to be selected as controls than those who are screened less frequently. With the proposed weighting a woman who is screened annually and would therefore always be eligible as a screened control would receive weight 1 whereas one who is screened every four years (and would only be eligible to be screened a quarter of the time, i.e. if one of her screens fell within the one-year interval in 2, above) would receive weight 4. This strategy would neutralise the bias in the extreme example above.

A final adjustment is necessary if screen-detected cancers are to be considered together with interval or sporadic cancers. The simplest approach is to normalise the weights so that the average weight given to each screened control is one.

Our definition of μ is not completely satisfactory particularly when $r = 0$. There is still a problem of how to define a routine smear and what to do when it is clear that a woman is being given multiple repeat smears. What for instance should be done about someone who has annual smears for five years following a single abnormal smear. If such a woman develops cancer and if she would without the abnormal smear have only had one smear every five years, then our analysis will give the impression that more frequent screening is associated with a greater risk of cervical cancer. This may be true, but the causality has been reversed. A woman who is at high risk of cancer is more likely to have a first abnormal smear, she is then more likely to have very frequent smear tests, so it is the cancer risk that causes the frequent screening rather than the reverse.

All methods that require controls for screen-detected cases to have been screened are subject to bias when there is some proportion of the population who are completely unscreened. This may not be immediately apparent since a screen-detected case would not be a case (until later) if she were completely unscreened. The problem arises when one tries to combine information from symptomatic and screen-detected cases. Suppose that 50% of women have three-yearly screening and 50% are unscreened. Suppose further that screening is of no benefit and that 50% of the cancers in the screened population will be screen detected. Then 2/3 of the symptomatic cancers will be in the unscreened women, whereas all of the screen-detected cancers will be in screened women. Using ordinary random controls for the symptomatic cases will yield a protective odds ratio of 2.0 for screening whereas using screened controls (weighted or unweighted) will give an odds ratio of 1.0 for the screen-detected cancers. It is clear then that it is also necessary to consider all cancers combined to demonstrate that screening is reducing the incidence of cancer. Screening may be beneficial even if it does not reduce the incidence of invasive cervical cancer, but that would require demonstration of a reduction in mortality or at least a reduction in the incidence of late-stage disease.

9.5 Statistical analysis

All case-control studies aimed at evaluating the effect of screening should be analysed by conditional logistic regression (Breslow and Day, 1980) since the controls should be individually matched to each case. At the very least matching should be performed on age, and the screening histories of a case and her control(s) should be curtailed on the date of diagnosis of the case's cancer. Failure to take account in the analysis of the matched design could cause serious bias in estimates of the screening effect.

9.6 Definition of exposure

We have discussed control selection at some length, but there remains the question of how to define exposure to screening. We need some measure of screening intensity and unfortunately this too is complicated. The simplest approach is to compare screened to unscreened women. This may work if there is no organised screening, but is likely to lack power if screening has been available for some years. Where screening is widely available, only a minority of the target population will be unscreened and these may be self-selected so that, even with the absence of a screening effect, their risk of cervical cancer may be quite different from that of women who participate in screening. For instance, nuns who may know that they are extremely low risk of developing cervical cancer may choose not to be screened; young women on the edge of society who are exposed to oncogenic HPV infection and are therefore at higher risk and have a subdued immune system (due to poor diet and drug abuse or even HIV infection) may be less likely to be screened. Thus differences in cancer incidence between screened and unscreened women may reflect factors influencing screening uptake rather than the effect of screening.

An extra problem arises in trying to distinguish screening from diagnostic smears. Although strictly speaking, smear tests play no part in the diagnosis of symptomatic cervical cancers, many doctors continue to take smears in women presenting with symptoms.

Thus it is common to find women in their 70s whose only smear was taken six weeks before the diagnosis of cancer. If a mildly dyskaryotic smear in a symptomatic woman is repeated at six months without colposcopy, the time from first (non-screening) smear to histological diagnosis of cancer could be up to nine months. It may be possible to distinguish between routine (screening) and symptomatic/diagnostic smears through a careful examination of clinical notes. For more routine case-control studies we suggest that all smears within several months of the date of cancer diagnosis be ignored in both the case and the controls. This prediagnosis period should be the same length for all individuals in a given health authority. It should be between 2 and 12 months depending on local policy and waiting times. Note, however, that negative smears taken just a few months prior to cancer diagnosis are of particular interest when studying cytology false negatives and should not be ignored for the purpose of laboratory audit.

Many case-control studies of cervical cancer have used the time since the last negative smear as the measure of screening intensity. This is a strange definition since a negative smear has never helped prevent cervical cancer. Analysis of the time to the last negative smear is useful because it provides information on the sensitivity of screening and the rate of cancer incidence following a negative test. In particular, sensitivity can be studied by comparing the relative risk of cancer x years after a negative smear in women who have had just one negative smear and in women who have had two or more (IARC, 1986). The decreased risk of cervical cancer in the years following a negative smear can be used to decide the frequency of screening, but it should not be used to estimate the benefit of screening. It is only after a non-negative smear result that a woman may be referred and treated for a precancerous lesion. The analysis of time since last negative screen does not take into account the chances that a woman with a non-negative screening test will be successfully treated. Some will never receive treatment and others, despite treatment, will develop invasive cancer.

Analysis of the time from the last negative smear is intended to provide information regarding the period of low risk following a negative smear. There is thus no need to exclude smears taken just before the date of cancer diagnosis. Indeed ignoring these could bias results by excluding a rare negative smear in a symptomatic woman.

What we are really interested in is some measure of the frequency with which a woman goes for screening. Unfortunately many case-control studies only have reliable screening data going back for a few years and the true screening interval may be difficult to estimate particularly if a woman has had several repeat smears following an abnormality. One approach is to use the measure μ defined earlier (in the subsection on weighted screened controls) as the individual's average screening interval. This has two disadvantages. Firstly, if a woman has just been screened, it should not (in theory) matter whether her previous smear was six months, two years or 10 years earlier, but the resulting μ's will be quite different. Secondly, if all women are screened exactly once in six years, this approach would have zero power to detect a screening effect. In general, if adherence to a strict screening interval is almost universal, there will be problems of insufficient variability to estimate effects.

An alternative strategy considers the time since the last adequate smear (excluding those within say six months of the date of the case's diagnosis) regardless of the smear result. In such an analysis it is desirable to try to distinguish smears that are taken as a result of a previous abnormality. The way in which this is done will depend on local policy. If smears are not repeated, then it may not be necessary to make an adjustment.

If abnormal smears are repeated at six-monthly intervals until two consecutive negatives or referral, then it may be sensible to exclude all smears taken in the 18 months (to allow for some delay in rescreening) following a non-negative adequate test result.

Analyses based on the time since the last smear can reasonably be used to estimate the protective effect if screening at a given interval. Once this has been done, the population attributable risk can be used to estimate the number of cases actually prevented by screening in the population being studied. This was done for a study in the UK (Sasieni et al., 1996).

9.7 Other practical considerations

9.7.1 Case identification

Where possible, cases should be identified from the regional Cancer Registry based on area of usual residence at the time of diagnosis. Where this is not possible or where there is substantial delay (or incompleteness) in the registration of cancers, cases can be identified from local pathology laboratories. Depending on the quality of the laboratory databases, one may also wish to contact gynaecological oncology departments. It is not considered necessary to go to great lengths to trace death-certificate-only cases since these will mostly be of an age at which they are unlikely to have been screened within the last 15 years.

In many regions it is difficult to accurately identify screen-detected cancers. One approach is to make a working definition based on the screening history – such a case must have had a smear warranting referral to colposcopy within three months of diagnosis. Another is to ignore the problem of the mode of presentation and instead distinguish between microinvasive (stage 1A) and fully invasive (stage 1B or worse) cancers. Such a minimal staging should be possible based on the histology report. Microinvasive cancers have extremely good prognosis and are generally without symptoms. Thus they may be considered as partial successes of screening. Fully invasive cancers, by contrast, are often fatal, require extensive surgery or radiotherapy and are rarely occult.

9.7.2 Screening histories

Traditional case-control studies use interviews and examination of GP notes to obtain the most accurate information on a woman's cervical screening history. Such labour-intensive research may not be feasible for regular monitoring or routine studies of cervical screening. In many regions a computerised call and recall population register stores the date and result of each smear taken on each woman. Where this is not available, local laboratories should be able to provide details on all smears from a given woman that they have analysed. The use of routine databases may break down when the population is extremely mobile so that a high proportion of women have had smears taken outside of the region over the past 5–10 years, but is likely to be cheap and accurate in other situations. It is suggested that the more labour-intensive approach be employed in addition to a routine method in a pilot study so that one can estimate the accuracy of the database approach within a given geographic area.

9.8 Conclusion

The problems considered in this paper are very real. The incidence of cervical cancer in the United Kingdom changed very little between 1975 and 1988 despite considerable cervical screening activity. This does not necessarily invalidate cervical screening and this chapter is not the place to discuss the reasons for the relatively static incidence rates. However, there is a great need to develop a method for routine analysis of screening programmes to estimate the potential beneficial effect of screening and to identify strengths and weaknesses of the current programme. In particular the issue of how frequently to screen is still not completely resolved. Many programmes have in place a computerised call and recall system that records the dates and results of every woman's cervical cytology test. This is an ideal resource for implementing an ongoing case-control study along the lines discussed in this chapter.

References

Bosch, F.X., Manos, M.M., Munoz, N., Sherman, M., Jansen, A.M., Peto, J. *et al.* (1995). Prevalence of human papillomavirus in cervical cancer: a worldwide perspective. International biological study on cervical cancer (IBSCC) Study Group [see comments]. *J. Natl. Cancer Inst.*, **87**, 796–802.

Breslow, N.E. and Day, N.E. (1980). *Statistical Methods in Cancer Research. Volume 1 – The Analysis of Case-control Studies.* International Agency for Research in Cancer, Lyon (IARC Scientific Publications No. 32).

Brisson, J., Bairati, I., Morin, C., Fortier, M., Bouchard, C., Christen, A. *et al.* (1996). Determinants, of persistent detection of human papillomavirus DNA in the uterine cervix. *J. Infect. Dis.*, **173**, 794–9.

Burk, R.D., Ho, G.Y., Beardsley, L., Lempa, M., Peters, M. and Bierman, R. (1996). Sexual behavior and partner characteristics are the predominant risk factors for genital human papillomavirus infection in young women. *J. Infect. Dis.*, **174**, 679–89.

Campion, M.J., McCance, D.J., Cuzick, J. and Singer, A. (1986). Progressive potential of mild cervical atypia: prospective cytological, colposcopic and virological study. *Lancet*, **2**, 237–40.

Cox, D.R. (1962). *Renewal Theory.* Chapman and Hall, London.

Cullen, A.P., Reid, R., Campion, M. and Lorincz, A.T. (1991). Analysis of the physical state of different human papillomavirus DNAs in intraepithelial and invasive cervical neoplasm. *J. Virol.*, **65**, 606–12.

Cuzick, J. (1997). Viral load as a surrogate for persistence in cervical human papillomavirus infection. In: Franco, E.L.F. and Monsonégo, J. (eds). *New Developments in Cervical Cancer Screening and Prevention.* Blackwell Science, Oxford, pp. 373–8.

Das, B.C., Sharma, J.K., Gopalakrishna, V. and Luthra, U.K. (1992). Analysis by polymerase chain reaction of the physical state of human papillomavirus type 16 DNA in cervical preneoplastic and neoplastic lesions. *J. Gen. Virol.*, **73**, 2327–36.

Dillner, J., Kallings, I., Brihmer, C., Sikstrom, B., Koskela, P., Lehtinen, M. *et al.* (1996). Seropositivities to human papillomavirus types 16, 18, or 33 capsids and to Chlamydia trachomatis are markers of sexual behavior. *J. Infect. Dis.*, **173**, 1394–8.

Evans, J., Redburn, J. and Roche, M. (1997). *Cervical Cancer in Berkshire, Buckinghamshire, Northamptonshire and Oxfordshire*. Oxford Cancer Intelligence Unit.

Herbert, A. and Smith, J.A.E. (1999). Cervical intraepithelial neoplasia grade III (CINIII) and invasive cervical carcinoma: the yawning gap revisited and the treatment of risk. *Cytopathology*, **10**, 161–70.

Hildesheim, A., Schiffman, M.H., Gravitt, P.E., Glass, A.G., Greer, C.E., Zhang, T. *et al.* (1994). Persistence of type-specific human papillomavirus infection among cytologically normal women [see comments]. *J. Infect. Dis.*, **169**, 235–40.

Ho, G.Y., Burk, R.D., Klein, S., Kadish, A.S., Chang, C.J., Palan, P. *et al.* (1995). Persistent genital human papillomavirus infection as a risk factor for persistent cervical dysplasia [see comments]. *Journal of the National Cancer Institute*, **87**, 1365–71.

IARC working group on the evaluation of cervical cancer screening programmes (1986). Screening for squamous cervical cancer: duration of low risk after negative results of cervical cytology and its implication for screening policies. *BMJ*, **293**, 659–64.

Kiviat, N.B., Critchlow, C.W. and Kurman, R.J. (1992). Reassessment of the morphological continuum of cervical intraepithelial lesions: does it reflect different stages in the progression to cervical carcinoma? In: Munoz, N., Bosch, F.X., Shah, K.V. and Meheus, A. (eds), *The Epidemiology of Cervical Cancer and Human Papillomavirus* (IARC Scientific Publications No. 119), IARC, Lyon, pp. 59–66.

Korobowicz, E., Kwasniewska, A. and Georgiades, I. (1997). The diagnostic value of cyto-morphological traits in low and high risk type HPV infections. *Polish Journal of Pathology*, **48**, 107–12.

Koutsky, L.A., Holmes, K.K., Critchlow, C.W., Stevens, C.E., Paavonen, J., Beckmann, A.M. *et al.* (1992). A cohort study of the risk of cervical intraepithelial neoplasia grade 2 or 3 in relation to papillomavirus infection. *New England Journal of Medicine*, **327**, 1272–8.

Miller, B.A., Ries, L.A.G., Hankey, B.F. *et al.* (eds). (1993). *SEER Cancer Statistics Review: 1973–1990*. National Cancer Institute. NIH Pub. No. 93–2789.

Office of National Statistics. (1998). *Registrations of Cancer Diagnosed in 1992, England and Wales*. Her Majesty's Stationery Office, London.

Ostor, A.G. (1993). Natural history of cervical intrepithelial neoplasia – a critical review. *Int. J. Gynecol. Pathol.*, **12**, 186–92.

Remmink, A.J., Walboomers, J.M., Helmerhorst, T.J., Voorhorst, F.J., Rozendaal, L., Risse, E.K. *et al.* (1995). The presence of persistent high-risk HPV genotypes in dysplastic cervical lesions is associated with progressive disease: natural history up to 36 months. *International Journal of Cancer*, **61**, 306–11.

Sasieni, P.D., Cuzick, J. and Lynch-Farmery, E. (1996). Estimating the efficacy of screening by auditing smear histories of women with and without cervical cancer. The National Co-ordinating Network for Cervical Screening Working Group. *Br. J. Cancer*, **73**, 1001–5.

van Ballegooijen, M., Akker, M.E. van den, Warmerdam, P.G., Meijer, C.J.L.M., Walboomers, J.M.M. and Habbema, J.D.F. (1997). Present evidence on the value of HPV testing for cervical cancer screening: a model-based exploration of the (cost-)effectiveness. *Br. J. Cancer*, **76**, 651–7.

Wheeler, C.M., Greer, C.E., Becker, T.M., Hunt, W.C., Anderson, S.M. and Manos, M.M. (1996). Short-term fluctuations in the detection of cervical human papillomavirus DNA. *Obstetrics and Gynecology*, **88**, 261–8.

10

Interpretation of the effect of population screening using routine incidence and mortality data

Timo Hakulinen

10.1 Introduction

It would be ideal if population-based mass-screening activities could always be evaluated as controlled trials. Unfortunately, this is not always possible as screening has in the past been considered as a pure service activity (Hakama, 1982). Even if proper trials have been conducted, it is possible that service screening will differ from screening in a trial in its quality and hence in its effectiveness. For example, compromises may be necessary in service screening, and the enthusiasm of the field staff may be lower in service screening compared to in a trial. Thus, it is important that an evaluation can be made of the screening activity even when a specific trial has not been designed. This kind of evaluation is an important component of quality assurance of any on-going screening programme.

It is natural that routine statistics on cancer mortality and incidence could be used for evaluation purposes. The main and ultimate indicator of the success of a screening programme is a decrease in mortality from the cancer in question. Changes in cancer incidence may be utilised if the cancer has a sufficiently long preclinical phase and if the treatment of a preinvasive lesion precludes its development into a truly invasive cancer. For example, cervical cancer has such a preinvasive stage while *in situ* lesions of the breast are less well defined and probably infrequent. Thus, in breast-cancer screening, mostly invasive but preclinical lesions are diagnosed in order to decrease breast-cancer mortality.

10.2 Design questions

A prerequisite for an empirical evaluation is a difference in screening policy. It may occur over time (Gibson *et al.*, 1997), and it may also exist between different geographical regions (Törnberg *et al.*, 1994). These differences should subsequently be reflected in differences in the temporal and geographical patterns of disease incidence or mortality. Thus, consistent and comparable information on disease occurrence and death should also exist.

The early examples on the evaluation of cervical-cancer screening using the Nordic data on incidence and mortality were rather clear-cut: in Norway screening was introduced much later than in the other Nordic countries, and both the cervical-cancer incidence and mortality had a clearly unfavourable course in Norway compared to the other Nordic countries (Figures 10.1 and 10.2).

It would be very important for a successful evaluation of a public health policy if the policy could be specifically designed to facilitate the evaluation. Finnish breast-cancer screening (Figure 10.3) provides a good practical example. As it was not possible, for practical reasons and due to lack of funding, to provide the screening service for everyone at the same time, a national recommendation was to start screening cohorts born in even years earlier than those born in odd years (Hakama *et al.*, 1997). A non-significant 24% reduction in breast-cancer mortality, based on the incident breast-cancer cases in the period 1987–92, was observed for the birth cohorts screened early, compared to those

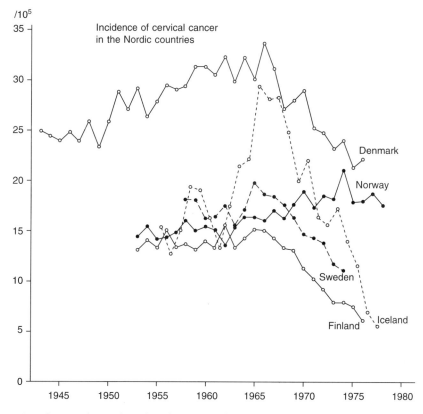

Figure 10.1 The annual age-adjusted incidence rates of cervical cancer in the Nordic countries in 1943–78 (Hakama, 1982)

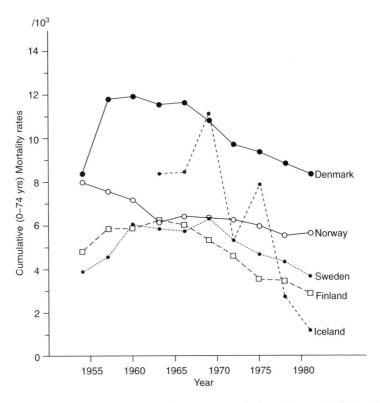

Figure 10.2 Triannual cumulative mortality rates (ages 0–74 years) of cervical cancer in the Nordic countries in 1953–82 (Läärä *et al.*, 1987)

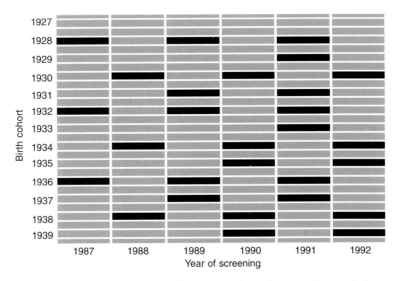

Figure 10.3 Finnish National Board of Health's recommendation for screening rounds in an organised programme for breast cancer, by birth cohort and calendar year (Hakama *et al.*, 1997)

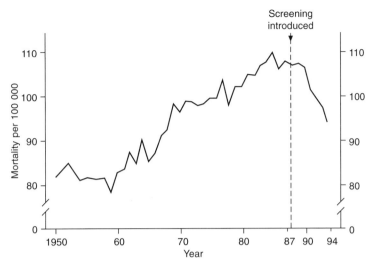

Figure 10.4 Age-adjusted mortality rates from breast cancer in women aged 55–69 years in England and Wales in 1950–94 (Quinn and Allen, 1995)

screened later. The reduction was 44% and significant among women aged under 56 years of age at the beginning of the study.

There may be confounders that may severely complicate the evaluation of a screening policy, unless there is a planned design as above or there are documented differences in the screening policy that could be regarded as a non-experimental design for a study. For example, treatment as a potential confounding factor should be controlled for when evaluating mammographic screening based on routine mortality data (Figure 10.4). Treatment with tamoxifen was widely adopted approximately at the same time when mammographic screening was introduced (Quinn and Allen, 1995). Thus, it became practically impossible to distinguish an independent effect of the screening.

10.3 Accounting for existing trends

It is important to take into account that the incidence and mortality rates may have existing trends and differentials that prevailed already before the screening activity started. Moreover, the areas may be internally heterogeneous with respect to disease trends and differentials. These factors should be taken appropriately into account when using a statistical model for the incidence or mortality. An appropriate model which has been built using that part of the incidence or mortality data that is not related to a time period when screening was practised may be extrapolated into the period of screening in order to give a theoretical expected number of cases or deaths in the absence of screening (Prior et al., 1996; Gibson et al., 1997). If the true observed number of cases or deaths is sufficiently below the expected one, screening may be considered successful. Information on the coverage or other aspects of the screening activity may be incorporated in the modelling in order to give a more detailed numerical effect of the screening (Törnberg et al., 1994).

When extrapolating trends, particular attention should be paid to technical aspects that may affect trends in cancer incidence and mortality (Hakulinen, 1996). Definitions and diagnostic criteria and facilities change over time and may make or mask trends. It may in principle be difficult to predict for how long these changes may continue. One might actually expect existing trends to level off in a curvilinear manner in the absence of further interventions such as screening. If mortality from a disease is declining, one could not reasonably expect it to continue to do so unless existing trends in therapy or stage at presentation also continue.

10.4 Statistical aspects

Building of a statistical model should be considered as a tailor-made activity for the particular problem at hand. The models employed in the comparisons are usually based on Poisson regression (Breslow and Day, 1987). They should take into account the uncertainty in the model parameters related to the randomness in the historical data and the random variability of the observations that are made in the period of the evaluation (Hakulinen and Dyba, 1994; Gibson et al., 1997).

Confidence intervals describe the range of likely outcomes under the assumption that the model that has been chosen is correct. A confidence interval (the middle intervals of the predictions in Figure 10.5) is actually built in such a way that only the uncertainty in the historical data is accounted for. A prediction interval (the total intervals of the predictions in Figure 10.5) also accounts for uncertainty in the future number of cases itself. Thus, the prediction intervals are somewhat wider than the corresponding confidence intervals.

If screening for melanoma and cancers of the colon, stomach or lung could be based on early detection of preclinical lesions and if such a screening had been started for one of the cancers in Figure 10.5 after 1980–85, one simple way to attempt to evaluate its effect would be to check whether the observed number in 2000–04 falls below the prediction intervals. Special attention should be given to possible confounding and other technical factors which may be involved.

Screening is usually targeted on certain age groups. When comparing the observed numbers with those predicted, it is useful to check that the effect is where it has been expected to be. The age-specific predicted and observed numbers for the incidence of breast cancer in Finland in 1989–93 agreed fairly well, with one major exception, given that the prediction base was 1954–83 (Figure 10.6), when there was no mammographic screening in Finland. In the years following the prediction base there was mammographic screening in ages 50–64 years, and indeed the observed numbers of new breast-cancer cases exceeded those predicted in those ages. The increased incidence is not beneficial per se but it should be in the years after the start of screening, as a result, among other possibilities, of an advancement of breast-cancer diagnoses. This in turn may lead to a decrease in breast-cancer mortality attributable to a lower fatality of these early detected tumours (Hakama et al., 1997).

If desired, it is also possible to use models that preserve the age-incidence pattern of the disease incidence in the period of prediction when calculating the theoretical expected or predicted numbers in the absence of screening (Dyba et al., 1997). Instead of using observed and expected numbers, the screening variable can be also explicitly included in the model either as an indicator (Luostarinen et al., 1995) or as a more sophisticated

Example 111

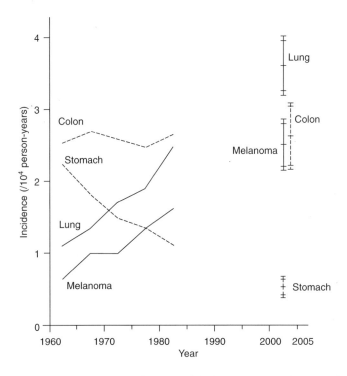

Figure 10.5 Age-adjusted incidence rates of cancers of the lung, stomach and colon and of melanoma of the skin in females in the Stockholm–Gotland Oncological Region in Sweden in 1960–84, by five-year period, with predictions for 2000–04: total interval: approximate 95% prediction interval for the future observation; the middle interval: 95% confidence interval for the expected value of the future observation (Hakulinen and Dyba, 1994)

screening score (Törnberg *et al.*, 1994). This not only facilitates and increases the efficiency of formal testing of the effect of the screening programme, but also helps in estimating its effect. An example of this is now given.

10.5 Example

This example comes from Törnberg *et al.* (1994). In the Swedish national guidelines on mammographic screening there were no instructions about the evaluation of service screening. Evidently, the assumption was that the screening would as a routine activity be as successful as the Swedish mammographic screening trials (Rutqvist *et al.*, 1990). Thus it was of interest, for future quality assurance, to check whether the effect of the large Swedish trials could be seen using routine breast-cancer mortality data and details about the screening.

The point of departure for the assessment was that the screening will reduce the breast-cancer mortality from a predicted level, based solely on trend extrapolation. In a given time interval, here a five-year period, however, a large part of breast-cancer mortality could still be related to cases diagnosed in an earlier period, potentially before the screening

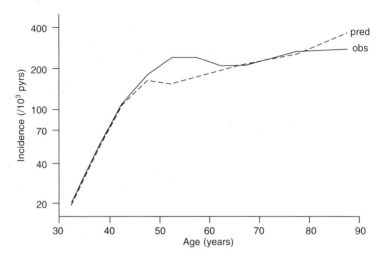

Figure 10.6 The predicted age-specific breast-cancer incidence in Finnish females (pred) and that observed (obs) in 1989–93, by age (Hakulinen, 1996)

was started. This was accounted for in the statistical model by assuming that the full effect of screening, whatever reduction it is, can only be seen starting from 10 years after the period in which the screening was initiated. In the preceding period, from 5 to 10 years after the initiation, the effect was assumed to be only half of that size, owing to cases diagnosed before the screening dying in that period. No effect was assumed to be observed during the first five years after the initiation of the screening programme.

The 26 Swedish counties were used as geographical units in the evaluation. Gävleborg county with a long history of service screening was excluded from this exercise. The age groups considered were those of the screening, five-year categories between 50 and 75 years. When only a proportion of an age group was subject to screening the effect of the programme on mortality was assumed to concern the proportion screened, only. For example, in Stockholm, the screening started in 1981 and covered 16% of the target population. Thus, in the first five years after the start of screening no reduction would be expected compared with the trend extrapolation. During 5–10 years after screening there would be 50% of a potential but unknown full reduction for 16% of the population, i.e. an 8% fraction of the full unknown reduction for the population of the whole of Stockholm. After 10 years there would be a full unknown reduction for 16% of the population, i.e. a 16% fraction of the full unknown reduction for the population.

If the trend extrapolation gave a predicted mortality of $60/10^5$ person-years for a period of analysis and if the full reduction due to mammographic screening were 33% (1/3), the expected mortality in a period 10 years or more after the screening started would be $(60 - 60/3)/10^5 = 40/10^5$. But if the program only concerned a (representative) fraction of 16% of the population, the reduction would be 16% of the expected reduction, i.e. $0.16 \times 20/10^5 = 3.2/10^5$, and the reduced mortality would be approximately $(60 - 3)/10^5 = 57/10^5$. The reduction would be only half of $3.2/10^5$ if the time period were located between 5 and 10 years after the start of screening.

Breast-cancer mortality was studied in five-year time periods between 1971 and 1990. There was no county with predicted deviations from mortality trends in the first two of

Table 10.1 Fractions of theoretical maximum effects (mammography scores) for the Swedish counties with mammographic screening trials in 1981–90 (Törnberg *et al.*, 1994)

County	Period	
	1981–85	1986–90
Stockholm	0	0.08
Östergötland	0.15	0.40
Malmö	0.25	0.50
Gothenburg	0	0.15
Kopparberg	0.27	0.60

the four time periods. In the last two periods, however, there were predicted deviations (Table 10.1). For example as stated above, Stockholm would experience an 8% fraction of the theoretical maximum reduction compared with the trend in 1986–90. The expected reduction was largest, 60% of the maximum effect, in Kopparberg in 1986–90. These fractions were called mammographic scores.

A Poisson regression model including the main effects of categorical age and period and of numerical mammography score gave a satisfactory fit to the breast-cancer mortality data. The *p*-value for removing the mammography score from the model was 0.08. The point estimate for the mammography score indicated a 19% protective effect, with 95% confidence interval ranging from –3% to 37%. There was no evidence that the effect of mammography score would have been different for different counties.

The 19% protective effect, even if non-significant, is in line with the 24% effect obtained in an overview of the Swedish trials (Nyström *et al.*, 1993). The modelling based on routine mortality data is naturally a cruder alternative than a proper evaluation of the trials. On the other hand, it is good to know that an effect can be found also in routine data when modelling has been done. But when such data are used to model service screening activity, it can be expected that the effects may end up being somewhat underestimated depending on the appropriateness of the model and on long-term survival of cases diagnosed a long time ago.

It was important that the trend extrapolations were based on a simultaneous modelling of the rates in all counties, and not on making a model for each county separately. When the number of counties is large, multi-level modelling can be used as an alternative (Rice and Leyland, 1996; Gibson *et al.*, 1997). With this method, the solutions become in practice more complex (e.g. Markov chain Monte Carlo technique, Gibbs sampling) than with the classical stratified fixed-effect Poisson regression techniques outlined above. On the other hand, extra mortality in the predicted rates caused by variability between regions may be more appropriately accounted for.

References

Breslow, N.E. and Day, N.E. (1987). *Statistical Methods in Cancer Research. Volume II. The Design and Analysis of Cohort Studies. IARC Scientific Publications No. 82.* International Agency for Research on Cancer, Lyon.

Dyba, T., Hakulinen, T. and Päivärinta, L. (1997). A simple non-linear model in incidence prediction. *Stat. Med.*, **16**, 2297–309.

Gibson, L., Spiegelhalter, D.J., Camilleri-Ferrante, C. and Day, N.E. (1997). Trends in invasive cervical cancer incidence in East Anglia from 1971 to 1993. *J. Med. Screen.*, **4**, 44–8.

Hakama, M. (1982). Trends in the incidence of cervical cancer in the Nordic countries. In: Magnus, K. (ed.) *Trends in Cancer Incidence. Causes and Practical Implications.* Hemisphere, Washington, pp. 279–92.

Hakama, M., Pukkala, E., Heikkilä, M. and Kallio, M. (1997). Effectiveness of the public health policy for breast cancer screening in Finland: population based cohort study. *Brit. Med. J.* **314**, 864–7.

Hakulinen, T. (1996). The future cancer burden as a study subject. *Acta Oncol.*, **35**, 665–70.

Hakulinen, T. and Dyba, T. (1994). Precision of incidence predictions based on Poisson distributed observations. *Stat. Med.*, **13**, 1513–23.

Läärä, E., Day, N.E. and Hakama, M. (1987). Trends in mortality from cervical cancer in the Nordic countries: association with organised screening programmes. *Lancet*, **I**, 1247–9.

Luostarinen, T., Hakulinen, T. and Pukkala, E. (1995). Cancer risk following a community-based programme to prevent cardiovascular diseases. *Int. J. Epidemiol.*, **24**, 1094–9.

Nyström, L., Rutqvist, L.E., Wall, S., Lindgren, A., Lindqvist, M., Rydén, S., Andersson, I., Bjurstam, N., Fagerberg, J., Frisell, J., Tabar, L. and Larsson, L.G. (1993). Breast cancer screening with mammography: overview of Swedish randomised trials. *Lancet*, **341**, 973–8.

Prior, P., Woodman, C.B.J., Wilson, S. and Threlfall, A.G. (1996). Reliability of underlying incidence rates for estimating the effect and efficacy of screening for breast cancer. *J. Med. Screen.*, **3**, 119–22.

Quinn, M. and Allen, E. (1995). Changes in incidence of and mortality from breast cancer in England and Wales since introduction of screening. *Brit. Med. J.*, **311**, 1391–5.

Rice, N. and Leyland, A. (1996). Multilevel models: applications to health data. *J. Health Serv. Res. Pol.*, **1**, 154–64.

Rutqvist, L.E., Miller, A.B., Andersson, I., Hakama, M., Hakulinen, T., Sigfússon, B.F. and Tabar, L. (1990). Chapter IV. Reduced breast-cancer mortality with mammography screening – an assessment of currently available data. *Int. J. Cancer*, Suppl., **5**, 76–84.

Törnberg, S., Carstensen, J., Hakulinen, T., Lenner, P., Hatschek, T. and Lundgren, B. (1994). Evaluation of the effect on breast cancer mortality of population based mammography screening programmes. *J. Med. Screen.*, **1**, 184–7.

11

Optimal use of Pap smear screening for cervical cancer

Stephen D. Walter

11.1 Introduction

The cervical Pap smear is widely used, but recommendations on whom should be screened and how often have varied considerably. Optimal use of the Pap smear depends on an understanding of the natural history of cervical cancer, in particular the length of its preclinical, screen-detectable phase (PCDP) and the test sensitivity. The PCDP refers to the time period during which the disease is potentially detectable by screening, if it is used; it comprises a period of preinvasive disease followed by an invasive phase. This paper uses a model of some case-control data on Pap smear screening histories to estimate parameters that reflect the duration of the PCDP and the test sensitivity. One can then predict the proportion of cervical cancer cases that may be detected by screening at various frequencies.

Although use of the Pap smear is widespread, it has never been evaluated in a randomised trial. Effectiveness has been inferred from observational data, including time trends and ecological comparisons (Parkin, 1997; Läärä *et al.*, 1987; Pettersen *et al.*, 1985; Walton *et al.*, 1982; Duguid *et al.*, 1985; MacGregor and Teper, 1978), and a limited number of cohort studies (Stenkvist *et al.*, 1984; Lynge and Poll, 1986; Boyes *et al.*, 1982). Certain practical difficulties complicate the reliable determination of cervical cancer incidence, including variability in reading cervical cytology specimens (Brown and Brown, 1986; Kato *et al.*, 1995; Fleming, 1997) and the imperfect correspondence of cytology and histology results (Walker *et al.*, 1986). Variation over time in these factors might affect the time trend and ecologic data.

In recent years, several case-control studies on cervical cancer screening have been carried out (see Parkin, 1997). Their advantages, such as rapidity and relatively low cost, must be weighed against potential biases; methodologic concerns include biased self-selection into screening programmes, biased reporting of screening histories, misclassification of diagnostic tests as screening procedures, and the appropriate definition of cases and controls.

Differential self-selection into cancer screening programmes may be in either direction, in general. For breast cancer, women at higher risk are more likely to accept screening, whereas for cervical cancer the reverse is true. Substantial variation has been noted in cervical screening rates between various socioeconomic, racial and educational groups (US Department of Health and Human Services, 1985). In addition, cancer cases diagnosed at screening facilities may not fully represent the population disease experience. Population-based case-control studies are therefore to be preferred, because they have the best potential for determining the optimal periodicity of screening (Dubin *et al.*, 1987).

Sasco *et al.* (1986) have reviewed various choices of case and control groups for evaluation of screening. If, as with the Pap smear, the purpose is to detect disease in a preinvasive state, and thus reduce the incidence of invasive disease, then cases should be persons with incident invasive disease; their screening history should cover the period prior to the diagnosis, excluding tests that are part of the diagnostic process itself. Controls should be sampled from those alive at the time of diagnosis of the cases; their screening history consists of smears taken up to the time of diagnosis of the case (Sasco *et al.*, 1986).

In practice it is difficult to distinguish true 'screening' smears (taken in the absence of symptoms or other suspicion of disease) from smears precipitated by symptoms or carried out in response to earlier abnormal smears. Physician records of symptoms may be incomplete, and patient recall may be imperfect. An empirical way to deal with this is to exclude all case and control smears for a certain time period before the case diagnosis, although this may be at the expense of losing useful screening information. In general it is not clear whether the patient or physician data are to be preferred for this type of analysis (Walter *et al.*, 1988).

It has been suggested that cases detected by screening should be kept separate in the analysis, and that their controls should be chosen from among those screened negative at the time of the case diagnosis (Sasco *et al.*, 1986). The screening histories for this group should exclude the diagnostic smear for the case and the corresponding control smear. If the invasive component of the PCDP is relatively short, then the case-control relative frequencies of screening will be similar for interval cases (not detected by screening) and prevalent (screen-detected) cases. Both types of case and their controls may then be combined in the analysis. We did this in the analysis presented here, because previous results and our results suggested a long non-invasive PCDP.

An IARC working group carried out a meta-analysis of case-control and cohort data from eight countries (IARC Working Group on the Evaluation of Cervical Cancer Screening Programs, 1986). Higher protection was found for women with two or more negative smears, especially in the previous five years. Little difference in protection was found by screening annually versus every three years. The relative protection associated with two negative smears was at least eight for the first three years; some risk reduction persisted for 6–9 years, consistent with the view that some preinvasive lesions may exist for at least 10 years. Relative protection did not appear to depend on the woman's age. Several other analyses (Dunn and Martin, 1967; Kashgarian and Dunn, 1970; Day and Walter, 1986; Habbema *et al.*, 1985; Bos *et al.*, 1997; van Oortmarssen and Habbema, 1995) have also suggested a long PCDP.

The IARC group estimated that screening every three years could prevent 91% of incident cases, and that 84% could be prevented by screening every five years. The optimum recommended frequency of screening has, however, been controversial. For example the American Cancer Society recommends annual screening, or less frequently at the discretion of a physician after three normal examinations (Fink, 1988). A Canadian workshop recommended screening every three years after two negative smears taken a year apart (Miller *et al.*, 1991). Others have suggested a longer screening interval, such as five years (van Ballegooijen *et al.*, 1992). Hakama reports that screening in Finland is actually repeated only every five years (Hakama and Louhivuori, 1988).

The analysis presented in this paper addresses the question of optimal usage of the Pap smear, using augmented data from the first published case-control study on cervical screening. After adopting an explanatory model of the screening process, the PCDP duration and test sensitivity will be estimated, and then used to predict the relative benefits of alternative screening strategies. The survival benefit accruing to screen-detected cases will also be discussed, based on a recent follow-up of the original study participants.

11.2 Methods

The cases in this study were Toronto residents aged 20–69 years with newly diagnosed invasive squamous cell carcinoma of the cervix (Clarke and Anderson, 1979). They were matched to five controls each on age, neighbourhood and type of dwelling. Participants were interviewed on their use of Pap smears, including the reasons for visits to the physician, the type of examination performed and relevant symptoms. All attending physicians were contacted to provide independent information regarding the dates of smears, the reasons they were taken, and the results. The results of the smears were generally reported according to Papanicolaou's original classification, the system in widespread use at the time of the study. The patients represent more than 80% of newly diagnosed cases in the base population during the study period. The survival status of the cases was updated to 1994 (yielding up to 18 years of follow-up since diagnosis), in order to compare the survival of screen-detected and clinically detected cases.

In order to investigate the completeness and quality of the data, we assessed the levels of patient–physician agreement. Comparisons were made between the interview data and physicians' records with respect to the existence of previous Pap smears, their timing, symptoms or other reason for taking the smear, and the clinical results.

Because of the difficulties of distinguishing true screening smears from those taken because of symptoms or suspicion of disease, or as part of the diagnostic process, we established several alternative rules for excluding smears, based on when they occurred, or because of a previous abnormal smear (see Table 11.1). An abnormal smear was defined as a Pap class 3, i.e. moderate, mild to moderate, or severe dysplasia, class 3 unspecified, or worse.

The basis for rule 1 is to eliminate smears taken as part of the diagnostic work-up of cases; the same exclusion is applied to the controls, to avoid biasing the case-control

Table 11.1 Alternative rules for excluding non-screening Pap smears

Rule 1:	Exclude all smears within three months of the diagnosis of cases, or within three months of the corresponding assigned date for the matched controls.
Rule 2:	Exclude the first abnormal smear (if any) and any subsequent smear for all women.
Rule 3:	Rules 1 and 2 combined: i.e. exclude all smears within three months of the diagnosis and also exclude the first abnormal smear and any subsequent smears.

comparison. Rule 2 (similar to that used by McGregor *et al.*, 1985) has the following rationale. Women with no smears or all normal smears show no evidence *from their screening data* that they had ever had cancer. For women with an abnormal smear some time before diagnosis, there are three possibilities: (i) the abnormal result was a false positive; (ii) it was a true positive, but the disease had subsequently regressed; or (iii) it was a true positive, but without regression. In case (iii), the date of the smear would estimate the time of disease onset earlier (and more accurately) than the 'official' date of diagnosis. The three possibilities cannot be distinguished for an individual patient. However, cases (i) and (ii) are more likely for women who had an abnormal smear followed by one or more normal smears before diagnosis occurred.

Rule 2 ignores some information from women with an abnormal smear before diagnosis, but the same exclusion is made in the control histories. If false positive results occur randomly with equal probability for cases and controls, then this exclusion rule should be unbiased. On the other hand, if some of the prediagnostic results are actually true positives, their suppression would increase the apparent length of the PCDP.

Rule 3 is a combination of rules 1 and 2. It tends to exclude the most smears, especially near to the time of diagnosis. This may tend to enhance the apparent benefit of screening, relative to rules 1 and 2.

Again because of the difficulty in identifying true screening smears (i.e. symptom-free), most of our analyses were done by including all smears, or by limiting the data to symptom-free smears only. Combining the three temporal exclusion rules with the two rules for symptomatology gives six possible analyses for each of the patient and physician data sets. Comparison of the results provides some useful insights into the interpretation of the data, and suggests the likely robustness of the conclusions.

11.3 Analysis

The data were first analysed by cross-tabulation of the case and control screening histories. Next, logistic regression was used with various characteristics of the screening history being introduced into the regressions in turn. The objective of this part of the analysis was to assess the importance of the intervals since and between screens, and aid the interpretation of the subsequent screening model analysis to estimate the PCDP and test sensitivity.

Details of the screening model, for use with prospective data or as modified to handle case-control data, have been given elsewhere (Walter and Day, 1983; Day and Walter, 1984; Brookmeyer *et al.*, 1986; Brookmeyer and Day, 1987). In brief, we take the incidence rate of interval cancers at time t, following screens at times $\{t_1, ..., t_n\}$, to be

$$I_n(t) = I^* \sum_{i=0}^{n} \beta^{n-i} \int_{t-t_{i+1}}^{t-t_i} f(y)\, dy \qquad (11.1)$$

where we define $t_0 = -\infty$ and $t_{n+1} = t$. I^* is the underlying incidence of cancer in the absence of screening; β represents the false negative rate of the screening test; and $f(y)$ is the p.d.f. of the sojourn time in the PCDP. Expression (11.1) indicates that the incidence at time t is a mixture of cases of varying duration, and who may have been screened various numbers of times. The shortest duration cases are those which have arisen since

t_n, and hence have never been screened; the next group is those whose duration is between $(t - t_n)$ and $(t - t_{n-1})$, and who have had one false negative screen result at time t_n. Cases of even longer duration may occur, with progressively increasing numbers of prior false negative screen results. The model can allow for some fraction of preclinical cases to be non-progressive, by specifying $f(y)$ to include a non-zero probability of the PCDP being infinite (or, in practical data analysis, as long as the maximum possible lifespan of the individual). Expression (11.1) is integrated between times t_i and t_{i+1} in order to obtain the expected incidence of interval cases for this time period, based on a given amount of person-time at risk.

The prevalence of screen-detected cancer among those screened at time t_n is given by

$$P_n = (1 - \beta)I^* \sum_{i=1}^{n} \beta^{n-i} \int_{t_n - t_i}^{\infty} \min[y - (t_n - t_i), t_i - t_{i-1}] f(y) \, dy \qquad (11.2)$$

Like (11.1), expression (11.2) is based on the notion that the prevalence at t_n involves a mixture of cases of varying lengths. Again, longer duration cases having progressively more false negative screening results in their history before their diagnosis occurs at the most recent screen.

In matched case-control data, we let H_{ij} be the screening history for the jth member of the matched set i (consisting of an incident case and R_i controls), with $j = 0$ specifically indicating the case. Let z be an indicator variable with values 0 for an incident case, and 2 for a control. The likelihood contribution for set i is

$$\frac{\Pr(H_{i0} \mid z = 0) \prod_{j=1}^{R_i} \Pr(H_{ij} \mid z = 2)}{\sum_{k=0}^{R_i} \Pr(H_{ik} \mid z = 0) \prod_{j \neq k} \Pr(H_{ij} \mid z = 2)}$$

which, after use of Bayes' theorem, simplification, and assuming that the disease incidence in the population is small, simplifies to

$$\frac{\Pr(z = 0 \mid H_{i0})}{\sum_{k=0}^{R_i} \Pr(z = 0 \mid H_{ik})} \qquad (11.3)$$

The probabilities $\Pr(z = 0|H)$ may be obtained from expression (11.1) for incidence, after suitable specification of the function $f(y)$.

For screen-detected cases, who are compared to controls screened at the same time, we follow a similar approach: H_{ij} represents the prior screening history of person j in the ith set, with $j = 1$ indicating the prevalent case member of the set, and $z = 1$ for the case. The likelihood contribution from the set is

$$\frac{\Pr(z = 1 \mid H_{i0})}{\sum_{k=0}^{R_i} \Pr(z = 1 \mid H_{ik})} \qquad (11.4)$$

The required probabilities in expression (11.4) may be derived from expression (11.2) for the expected prevalence, for a specified screening history and the function $f(y)$. The combined likelihood from expressions (11.3) and (11.4) over all matched sets is maximised to obtain maximum likelihood estimates of parameters describing the PCDP distribution and the test sensitivity. Results will be shown assuming an exponential form of $f(y)$, characterised by its mean value. Finally, the survival of screen-detected and interval cancer cases can be compared using standard life table methods, with a possible adjustment for lead time.

Note that for the incidence cases and their controls, one is effectively estimating the ratio of incidences for individuals with given screening histories, whereas for the screen-detected cases and their controls, one is estimating a corresponding ratio of disease prevalences. A pooled analysis of the incident and screen-detected cases is appropriate if these two case-control ratios of screening history are numerically similar, which will occur if the duration of invasive disease is short relative to the entire PCDP (Sasco *et al.*, 1986). As discussed previously, previous analyses have suggested a long PCDP for cervical cancer, so the adoption of a pooled analysis strategy seems reasonable here.

11.3.1 Available sample sizes

There were 181 cases and 703 controls with interview data on screening histories. Of these, 123 cases and 391 controls had sufficient data from all their physicians to construct the screening history from medical records. Both patient and physician data sets were used in the cross-tabulations and logistic regressions. However, the screening models were restricted to the physician data only, because the month of smears was not specifically requested in the interview schedule, and so exact months were not available in the patient data; also, the estimated model parameters are sensitive to small changes in the dates of smears relatively close to the time of diagnosis. To reduce bias, the model data were limited to the 110 matched sets where the case and at least one control had complete physician information on screening histories.

The main determinant of physician data being missing was the length of time since the last patient visit; data were often missing because of practical difficulty in locating the physician after a relatively long period. The response rate for physicians visited in the past year was over 90%, but for physicians not seen for at least 10 years the response rate was only 60%. The response rate did not depend on the number of physicians mentioned in the interview, and was similar for cases (88%) and controls (86%).

11.3.2 Patient–physician agreement

An analysis of the agreement between patients and their physicians has been published elsewhere (Walter *et al.*, 1988), but is summarised here. There was moderately good agreement on the frequency of Pap smears, the times when they occurred, and the smear results. Agreement was better when it was confined simply to 'ever/never' screened. Cases and controls both tended to over-report the number of recent Pap smears, probably because of memory telescoping. Patient reporting of dates was a little more accurate for the cancer cases than for controls.

More symptoms were reported during interviews than were documented in the physician records, but it is not clear which data source is more accurate. Disagreement on the clinical results of Pap smears was due in part to imprecise terminology used by patients; agreement was good when restricted to 'normal/abnormal' comparisons.

11.4 Results

Table 11.2 shows the numbers of cases and controls who were never or ever screened. Proportionally more cases than controls were never screened; the difference is more marked in the symptom-free data, using exclusion rules 2 and 3 as opposed to rule 1, and in the physician data. The lower effectiveness estimates with rule 1 are likely due to the inclusion of diagnostic smears taken before the three-month cut-off, especially when all smears are included.

Table 11.3 shows results from the logistic regression analyses considering the most recent smear (if any) in the physician file data. The dependent variable was coded to show the odds ratio of being a *control*: thus the odds ratios for 'ever screened' and 'time since last smear' show the *protection* of ever being screened and its dependence on the screening frequency. The protective effect is somewhat greater when the analysis is restricted to symptom-free smears, or when exclusion rules 2 and 3 are used. Results with rules 2 and 3 in the symptom-free data suggest that the protection decreases by about one-third for each additional year since the last smear. There was, however, no strong effect of the time since the last smear when all smears were included. Additional analyses showed that the effects of the second most recent smear were almost always non-significant. Very similar results were obtained from the corresponding patient data.

Table 11.4 shows the maximum likelihood estimates of the mean PCDP and the test sensitivity, derived from the screening model. In the analysis of all smears, the estimated

Table 11.2   Case-control comparison of screening status

			Cases		Controls		
Data source	Smears included	Exclusion rule	Never screened	Ever screened	Never screened	Ever screened	Odds ratio
MD	All	1	67	56	112	279	3.0 **
MD	All	2	70	53	103	288	3.7 **
MD	All	3	81	42	113	278	4.7 **
MD	SF	1	88	35	137	254	4.7 **
MD	SF	2	94	29	139	261	6.5 **
MD	SF	3	95	28	138	253	6.2 **
Patient	All	1	67	114	225	478	1.3 NS
Patient	All	2	100	81	212	491	2.9 **
Patient	All	3	111	70	226	477	3.3 **
Patient	SF	1	133	48	343	360	2.9 **
Patient	SF	2	137	44	337	366	3.4 **
Patient	SF	3	138	43	344	359	3.3 **

MD = physician; SF = symptom-free; ** $p < 0.01$; NS = non-significant

Table 11.3 Logistic regression results for case-control comparison of screening histories

Smears included	Smear exclusion rule	Odds ratio[†]	
		Ever screened	Time since last smear
All	1	2.41 **	1.17
	2	3.82 **	0.96
	3	6.17 **	0.83
Symptom-free	1	5.26 **	0.93
	2	12.94 **	0.65 **
	3	12.43 **	0.67 *

[†]Estimates refer to the odds of being a control, relative to the odds of being a case
*$p < 0.05$; ** $p < 0.01$

Table 11.4 Maximum likelihood estimates of mean preclinical duration and screening sensitivity (physician data)

Smears included	Estimate	Exclusion rule		
		1	2	3
All	Mean preclinical duration (yrs)	12.5	21.7	19.7
	Test sensitivity	0.53	0.64	0.77
Symptom-free	Mean preclinical duration (yrs)	14.0	13.0	13.7
	Test sensitivity	0.71	0.87	0.90

mean PCDP is shorter when rule 1 is applied. This is because some abnormal smears are then included in the screening histories, but effectively are regarded as false positive results; this puts a more recent bound on the date when the PCDP could have begun, and reduces its average length. There is also a corresponding fall in the test sensitivity. In contrast, the analyses using only the symptom-free smears give very similar estimates of the PCDP duration, regardless of which exclusion rule is used. This may be because the proportion of abnormal smear results is smaller for asymptomatic investigations.

Note also that the sensitivity in the symptom-free analysis is somewhat lower with rule 1. When abnormal smears are included (under rule 1), they probably include some 'true' abnormalities, but which were insufficient to establish a firm diagnosis of disease at the time. Including such smears in the screening history thus reduces the estimated sensitivity. When abnormal and subsequent smears are eliminated (with rules 2 and 3), sensitivity is higher for the smears that remain.

The same effect on sensitivity is apparent in the analysis of all smears, where the sensitivity is lower than the all-smears analysis with each of the three exclusion rules. This is again because the all-smears analysis will effectively count some true abnormalities as normal.

The model results can now be used to estimate the percentage of cases that would be screen-detected under various screening policies: see Day and Walter (1984) for details of the method. For simplicity we suppose that screening is carried out at regular intervals for a certain period of time. Table 11.5 shows the cumulative percentage of cervical cancer cases that would be screen-detected over a 10-year period, based on the PCDP duration and screen sensitivity estimates from Table 11.4, for various screening frequencies. There are only small differences between these estimates for the all-smears and symptom-free smears analyses, especially under rules 2 and 3. The most discrepant estimate is from the 'all-smears' analysis with exclusion rule 1, where the estimated effectiveness of screening is somewhat lower; here the estimated PCDP duration and sensitivity are lower than in the other analyses, implying that it would be more difficult for the screen to detect a high percentage of cases with a given screening effort. Given that the invasive period of cervical cancer is short relative to the total PCDP duration, most of the individuals estimated to benefit from screening will be detected before invasive disease has developed.

Note that a substantial screening benefit is achieved with only one Pap test in 10 years, and the marginal gains by screening twice or even five times as often are relatively small. This suggests that the most important objective of Pap smear screening programmes should be to encourage first-time attendance for screening.

The survival curves of 15 screen-detected and 165 clinically detected cancers are shown in Figure 11.1, up to the maximum of 18 years of follow-up available. Adopting a liberal approach, we defined cases to have been screen-detected for this purpose if there had been a screen within the previous 12 months with a grade 3 result or higher, and if there were no symptoms at the time of presentation. This definition is possibly generous to the screening programme, in the sense that some of these cases might actually have been interval cases.

The survival difference favoured the screen-detected group, with an approximately 20% difference persisting between 5 and 15 years of follow-up. However, the overall difference in these curves was not statistically significant (Wilcoxon test, $p = 0.13$). There were only six deaths in the screen-detected group, and so it was not meaningful to make a formal adjustment to the survival curve to allow for the lead time included in the survival of screen-detected cases (Walter and Stitt, 1987). Such an adjustment would, of course, tend to reduce the apparent benefit of screening seen in Figure 11.1.

Table 11.5 Cumulative percentage of cervical cancer cases detected by screening with various frequencies, over 10 years

Smears included	Inter-screening interval (yrs)	Total smears over 10 years	Cumulative percent screen-detected with smear exclusion rule		
			1	2	3
All	2	5	85	94	95
	5	2	69	86	89
	10	1	51	74	79
Symptom-free	2	5	92	94	95
	5	2	81	87	89
	10	1	67	74	77

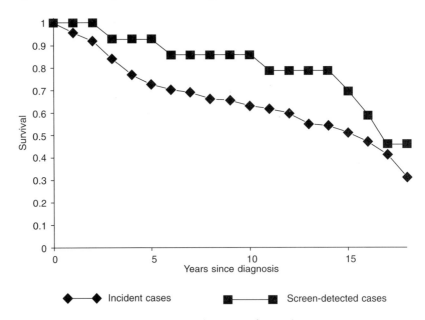

Figure 11.1 Survival of screen-detected and incident cases of cervical cancer

11.5 Conclusions

These analyses support the view that screening by the Pap smear is potentially capable of reducing mortality from cervical cancer. The long estimated PCDP and the high sensitivity of the test both indicate the attractiveness of this form of cancer prevention.

Greater protection associated with screening was suggested by the data derived from physician records and restricted to symptom-free smears, especially when abnormal smears and smears taken shortly before the diagnosis of the cases were excluded. The time since the last smear was also predictive of risk. The mean duration of preclinical screen-detectable disease was estimated to be approximately 14 years. Estimated test sensitivity was up to 90% when attention was restricted to symptom-free smears, and excluding prediagnostic smears. A non-significant survival advantage was noted for screen-detected cancer cases.

The analysis highlighted the difficulties of precisely identifying true screening smears. Despite some variation in the estimated parameter values according to which smears are counted as screens, the results clearly indicate that the greatest protection is associated with the first screen, with relatively little additional protection afforded by later smears. We estimate that approximately 90% of cervical cancer cases can be detected by screening once every five years. Most of the benefit is achieved with the first Pap smear; the additional advantage of screening more often than once every five years is rather small.

In a successful screening programme, the major benefit accrues by detecting disease cases in the preinvasive state, thus obviating the development of invasive disease. More frequent screening results in relatively more cases being identified preinvasively. In contrast, the survival advantage associated with screen-detection of disease that has already become invasive may be relatively small. This is reflected in our finding only a small difference in the survival of screen-detected and incident cases.

The priority for cervical screening programmes should therefore be to encourage first-time attendance, and to use strategies to increase compliance. The idea of encouraging more women to participate and increasing population coverage, rather than 'inviting the same women to attend more often' (Koopmanschap *et al.*, 1990) also has merit from the cost-effectiveness point of view.

Acknowledgements

Technical assistance in this project was provided by L.W. Stitt, A. Newman and J. Hatcher. The author thanks Dr E.A. Clarke for access to the original data from the Toronto study.

References

Bos, A.B., van Ballegooijen, M. and van Oortmarssen, G.J. *et al.* (1997). Non-progression of cervical intraepithelial neoplasia estimated from population-screening data. *Brit. J. Cancer*, **75**, 124–30.

Boyes, D.A., Morrison, B., Knox, E.G. *et al.* (1982). A cohort study of cervical cancer screening in British Columbia. *Clin. Invest. Med.*, **5**, 1–29.

Brookmeyer, R. and Day, N.E. (1987). Two-stage models for the analysis of cancer screening data. *Biometrics*, **43**, 657–70.

Brookmeyer, R., Day, N.E. and Moss, S. (1986). Case-control studies for estimation of the natural history of preclinical disease from screening data. *Stat. Med.*, **5**, 127–38.

Brown, L.J.R. and Brown, L. (1986). Cervical screening. *Lancet*, **2**, 925.

Clarke, E.A. and Anderson, T.W. (1979). Does screening by 'Pap' smears help prevent cervical cancer? A case-control study. *Lancet*, **2**, 1–4.

Day, N.E. and Walter, S.D. (1984). Simplified models of screening for chronic disease: estimation procedures for mass screening programs. *Biometrics*, **40**, 1–14.

Day, N.E. and Walter, S.D. (1986). Screening for cancer of the breast and cervix – estimating the duration of the detectable preclinical phase. In: Moolgavkar, S.H. and Prentice, R.L. (eds). *Modern Statistical Methods in Chronic Disease Epidemiology*, Wiley, New York.

Dubin, N., Friedman, D.R., Tonolio, P.G. *et al.* (1987). Breast cancer detection centers and case-control studies of the efficacy of screening. *J. Chronic Dis.*, **40**, 1041–50.

Duguid, H.L.D., Duncan, I.D. and Currie, J. (1985). Screening for cervical intraepithelial neoplasia in Dundee and Angus 1962–81 and its relation with invasive cervical cancer. *Lancet*, **2**, 1053–6.

Dunn, J.E. and Martin, P.L. (1967). Morphogenesis of cervical cancer. *Cancer*, **20**, 1899–906.

Fink, D.J. (1988). Change in American Cancer Society checkup guidelines for detection of cervical cancer. *CA – A Journal for Clinicians*, **38**, 127–8.

Fleming, K.A. (1997). Evidence-based pathology. *Evidence-Based Med.*, **2**, 132–3.

Habbema, J.D., van Oortmarssen, G.J., Lubbe, J.T. and van der Maas, P.J. (1985). Model building on the basis of Dutch cervical cancer screening data. *Mauritas*, **7**, 11–20.

Hakama, M. and Louhivuori, K. (1988). A screening programme for cervical cancer that worked. *Cancer Surveys*, **7**, 403–16.

IARC Working Group on the Evaluation of Cervical Cancer Screening Programs (1986). Screening for squamous cervical cancer: duration of low risk after negative results of cervical cytology and its implication for screening policies. *Brit. Med. J.*, **293**, 659–64.

Kashgarian, M. and Dunn, J.E. (1970). The duration of intraepithelial and preclinical squamous cell carcinoma of the uterine cervix. *Amer. J. Epidemiol.*, **92**, 211–22.

Kato, I., Santamaria, M., de Ruiz, P.A. *et al.* (1995). Inter-observer variation in cytological and histological diagnoses of cervical neoplasia and its epidemiologic implication. *J. Clin. Epidemiol.*, **48**, 1167–74.

Koopmanschap, M.A., van Ooortmarssen, G.J., van Agt, H.M. *et al.* (1990). Cervical-cancer screening: attendance and cost-effectiveness. *Int. J. Cancer*, **45**, 410–15.

Läärä, E., Day, N.E. and Hakama, M. (1987). Trends in mortality from cervical cancer in the Nordic countries. *Lancet*, **1**, 1247–9.

Lynge, E. and Poll, P. (1986). Incidence of cervical cancer following negative smear: a cohort study from Maribo County, Denmark. *Am. J. Epidemiol.*, **124**, 345–52.

MacGregor, J.E. and Teper, S. (1978). Mortality from carcinoma of the cervix uteri in Britain. *Lancet*, **2**, 774–6.

MacGregor, J.E., Moss, S.M., Parkin, D.M. *et al.* (1985). A case-control study of cervical cancer screening in north-east Scotland. *Brit. Med. J.*, **290**, 1543–6.

Miller, A.B. *et al.* (1991). Report of a National Workshop on screening for cancer of the cervix. *Canadian Med. Assoc. J.*, **145**, 1301–26.

Parkin, D.M. (1997). The epidemiological basis for evaluating screening policies. In Franco, E. and Monsonego, J. (eds) *New Developments in Cervical Cancer Screening and Prevention.* Blackwell, Oxford.

Pettersen, F., Bjorkholm, E. and Naslund, I. (1985). Evaluation of screening for cervical cancer in Sweden: trends in incidence and mortality 1958–80. *Int. J. Epidemiol.*, **14**, 521–7.

Sasco, A.J., Day, N.E. and Walter, S.D. (1986). Case-control studies for the evaluation of screening. *J. Chronic Dis.*, **9**, 399–405.

Stenkvist, B., Bergstrom, R., Eklund, G. *et al.* (1984). Papanicolaou smear screening and cervical cancer. What can you expect? *JAMA*, **252**, 1423–6.

US Department of Health and Human Services (1985). *Health Promotion and Disease Prevention US 1985: Data from National Health Survey.* Vital and Health Statistics, Series 10, 163. Bethesda.

van Ballegooijen, M., Habbema, J.D., van Oortmarssen, G.J. *et al.* (1992). Preventive Pap-smears: balancing costs, risks and benefits. *Brit. J. Cancer*, **65**, 930–3.

van Oortmarssen, G.J. and Habbema, J.D. (1995). Duration of preclinical cervical cancer and reduction in incidence of invasive cancer following negative Pap smears. *Int. J. Epidemiol.*, **24**, 300–7.

Walker, E.M., Dodgson, J. and Duncan, I.D. (1986). Does mild atypia on a cervical smear warrant further investigation? *Lancet*, **2**, 672–3.

Walter, S.D. and Day, N.E. (1983). Estimation of the duration of a preclinical disease state using screening data. *Amer. J. Epidemiol.*, **118**, 865–86.

Walter, S.D. and Stitt, L.W. (1987). Evaluating the survival of cancer cases detected by screening. *Stat. Med.*, **6**, 885–900.

Walter, S.D., Clarke, E.A., Hatcher, J. *et al.* (1988) A comparison of physician and patient reports of Pap smear histories. *J. Clin. Epidemiol.*, **41**, 401–10.

Walton, R.J. *et al.* (1982). Cervical cancer screening programs: summary of the 1982 Canadian Task Force Report. *Canadian Med. Assoc. J.*, **127**, 581–9.

12

Population-based breast cancer screening programmes: estimates of sensitivity, over-diagnosis and early prediction of the benefit

Eugenio Paci, Stephen W. Duffy, Daniela Giorgi,
Teresa C. Prevost and Marco Rosselli del Turco

12.1 Introduction

At the end of the 1980s a consensus emerged that mammographic screening could reduce mortality from breast cancer and several countries in Europe initiated population-based breast cancer screening programmes (van Ineveld *et al.*, 1993). Evaluation of regional and national programmes has been mainly through indicators of performance, such as detection rates, the proportion of small cancers among screen-detected cases and the rate of interval cancer incidence by time since the last negative test (Day *et al.*, 1989, 1995; Moss *et al.*, 1995; Tabar, 1995). These indicators are useful and it is extremely important that screening programmes are monitored for them and that the standards suggested for them are achieved. Nevertheless, such performance indicators are only partially able to predict the success of the screening programme (Tabar, 1995).

The primary aim of a population-based breast cancer screening programme is breast cancer mortality reduction, which is only observable with certainty some 8–10 years after the start of the programme. Also, evaluation of the impact of screening on breast cancer mortality over a period of time will invariably be complicated by the contemporaneous influence of other innovations, such as the introduction of better treatments for breast cancer. It is therefore useful to obtain early measures which are predictive of this final outcome and which are not confounded with changes in therapy.

In recent years the widespread practice of breast cancer early detection in clinical practice has occasioned, especially in the United States, an increase in breast cancer incidence in the general population and the detection of a large number of carcinomas *in situ* related to mammography (Ernster and Barclay, 1997). A temporary increase in the number of cases related to the increasing number of women taking up screening for breast cancer is to be expected and this increase is not necessarily an indicator of over-diagnosis. The excess depends on over-diagnosis, if any, on the sensitivity of screening and on the mean sojourn time (MST), the average duration of the period in which a tumour is asymptomatic but detectable by screening. A few years after the start of the programme, the number of cases occurring in the target population is expected to return approximately to the level expected in the absence of screening. Nevertheless, concern has been expressed that some of the excess incidence, notably of carcinoma *in situ*, may not be transient and may be a product of systematic over-diagnosis (Ernster and Barclay, 1997).

Population-based programmes need evaluation using markers able to be predictors of mortality. It has been shown that a good prediction of subsequent mortality can be made from the stage of disease or from a combination of tumour size, lymph node status and malignancy grade of the cancers diagnosed (Organizing Committee and Collaborators, 1996). A full evaluation should assess and take into account in prediction of mortality, the extent of over-diagnosis, if any.

In this chapter, we provide an example of the use of biostatistical and epidemiological methodology in evaluation of a population-based screening programme:

1. for the evaluation of over-diagnosis; and
2. for the prediction of mortality reduction.

The analysis is based on the results of the first two rounds of screening in the programme carried out in Florence, Italy.

12.2 The screening programme and data available

Women were enrolled from September 1990 until January 1993 (Figure 12.1). There were 53 579 receiving a first screening invitation in this period. Considering 1 January 1990 as the date of entry, all women were followed up for the occurrence of breast cancer up to the first screening invitation. Person-years at risk of incidence of breast cancer were estimated, and breast cancer cases diagnosed before first invitation date have been considered as the reference population (NYI, not-yet-invited). There were 116 715 person-years at risk before first invitation, and 270 invasive and 14 *in situ* carcinomas were observed. After the first screening invitation, the 53 579 invited women were categorised as responders (29 161, 54%) or non-responders (24 418, 46%) to the invitation. On average after 2.42 years, all women still resident in the area had been invited to the second screening round, and 21 504 attended. There were 235 cancers (214 invasive) diagnosed at the prevalence screen and 89 (74 invasive) at the incidence screen. There were 51 interval cancers (46 invasive) in the 2.42 years between the two screens.

Screen-detected breast cancer cases are those detected as a direct result of the mammography screening (at the first or repeated test); interval cancer cases are those detected within 2.42 years after a negative screening test. Breast cancer cases in those who did not attend the first screening round, diagnosed clinically before the second invitation, are classed as cases in non-responders (NRESP).

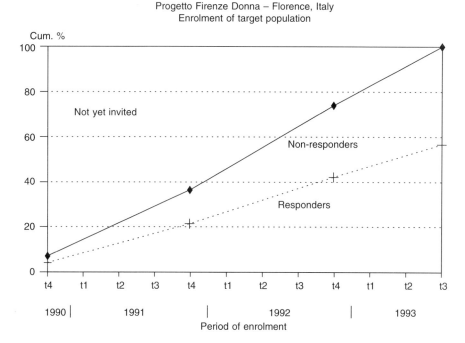

Figure 12.1 Enrolment by time in the Florence breast screening programme

12.3 Sensitivity, mean sojourn time and programme predictive value

Using the method of Prevost *et al.* (1998), we derived four sets of estimates of sensitivity (*S*) and MST. The four sets of estimates were derived by using either the prevalence screen or incidence screen cases for estimation (interval cancer cases were invariably used) and on whether the estimates were based on all tumours or on invasive tumours only. The assumptions involved are that incidence of preclinical disease and transition from preclinical to clinical disease both have exponential distributions with rates λ_1 and λ_2 respectively. λ_1 is approximately equal to the incidence of clinical cancer in the absence of screening, and in our case is estimated from the women not yet invited to screening. The MST can be estimated as $1/\lambda_2$. The expected number of breast cancer cases at the prevalence screen is

$$\frac{N_0 S \lambda_1}{\lambda_2}$$

The number of cases expected at the incidence screen is

$$\frac{S N_1 \lambda_1 (e^{-2.42\lambda_1} - e^{-2.42\lambda_2})}{\lambda_2 - \lambda_1} + \frac{N_0 S (1 - S) \lambda_1 e^{-2.42\lambda_2}}{\lambda_2}$$

where N_0 is the number attending the prevalence screen and N_1 the number attending the incidence screen. The first component of the expected number at incidence screen represents tumours newly incident in the preclinical detectable period since the prevalence screen and the second component represents those tumours missed at the prevalence screen. The 2.42 is the interscreening interval length in years in the Florence programme.

The ratio of the expected to the observed number of screen-detected cases is known as the positive predictive value (PPV) programme. A PPV of 100% or more means that the number of cases detected at screening is not in excess of that expected from the underlying incidence in the population, the progression rate of the disease and the sensitivity of screening. This in turn indicates that there is no evidence of over-diagnosis. A PPV of less than 100% will suggest that more cases are detected at the screening test than one would expect, and would be an indicator of possible over-diagnosis. For example, a PPV of 90% would suggest that 10% of the screen-detected cases would not have come to light clinically in the absence of screening and are therefore over-diagnosed.

12.4 Prediction of mortality reduction

Day and Duffy (1996) proposed to predict the effect of a screening regime on mortality by estimating the number of deaths from the prognostic attributes of the tumours diagnosed in a set of incident cancers in a screening programme, and comparing these with those estimated from a contemporaneous comparable group of incident tumours. They developed the methodology for purposes of comparison of two screening regimes, but the method is also valid for comparison of a group invited to screening with a contemporaneous uninvited group (in Florence, the NYI group).

In the context of a screening programme, a set of incident tumours consists of all cancers diagnosed from immediately after a negative screening test up to and including those diagnosed at the next screening test. This group is often referred to as the unbiased set, since it is largely free of length bias (Day and Duffy, 1996). When expressed as an incidence rate, it should be similar to the incidence in an uninvited group.

In order to compare the occurrence and fatality of cases in the unbiased set with the clinical incidence of breast cancer in women before the invitation (the NYI group), the possibility of selection bias between responders and non-responders to the invitation needs to be considered. The estimate of the total incidence based on the whole invited group (responders + non-responders) is unbiased. However, to estimate the impact of screening in the respondent group of women only, overcoming the diluting effect of the non-attendance, we have also estimated the expected number of cases correcting for differences in incidence between respondent and non-respondent women. This is done on the basis of the uninvited women containing unidentified populations of potential responders and non-responders in the same proportions and with the same incidence as in the invited group. The estimated incidence among the potential responders in the NYI group is

$$I_R = \frac{I_{NYI} - I_{NR}(1 - p)}{p}$$

where I_R is the estimated incidence in responders in the NYI group, I_{NYI} is the observed incidence in the NYI group, I_{NR} is the observed incidence in the non-responders in the invited group and p is the proportion of responders in the invited group.

The prediction of mortality at 10 years was based on the survival by UICC-pTNM staging (UICC, 1987). Fatality at 10 years was calculated from the 2468 tumours diagnosed in the Swedish Two-County Study (Tabar *et al.*, 1995), as 0.0713 for stage 1 or *in situ* tumours, 0.4156 for tumours at stage II+ and 0.3213 for tumours with stage unknown.

The predicted relative mortality is the ratio of the rate of deaths per person-year in the invited compared to the non-invited group. The 95% confidence interval was calculated using the formula of Day and Duffy (1996).

12.5 Results

Incidence of all cancers in the NYI group was 2.43 per thousand person-years (284/116 715). Incidence of invasive cancers was 2.31 per thousand (270/116 715). Table 12.1 shows the estimates of sensitivity and MST stratified by whether *in situ* tumours were used and which screen (incidence or prevalence) was used. The advantage of having one set estimated using the incidence screen and another using the prevalence is that we can then estimate the predictive value for one screen using the estimates from the other.

The expected number of cases (invasive and *in situ*) at the prevalence screen is calculated using the first column of Table 12.1(b) as:

$$\frac{N_0 S \lambda_1}{\lambda_2} = \frac{29\,161 \times 0.94 \times 0.00243}{1/3.75} = 250$$

Compared to the observed 235 tumours, this gives a PPV in excess of 100%, suggesting no over-diagnosis. When invasive tumours alone are considered, we expect 244 invasive cancers, compared to the 214 observed, again showing no indication of over-diagnosis. The number of *in situ* carcinomas observed was 21 versus the expected number of 6 (250 – 244). There is therefore a deficit of 30 invasive cases and an excess of 15 *in situ* at prevalence screen.

Using the figures in Table 12.1(a) and the more complex formula for expected cases at the incidence screen, we estimate an expected total number of invasive and *in situ* cases at the incidence screen of 95, versus the 89 observed. For invasive cancers only, we expect 84, compared to the 74 observed. Thus, again, there is no evidence of over-diagnosis; indeed the observed number of cancers is smaller than expected. There is a deficit of 10 invasive tumours and an excess of 4 *in situ* (15 observed compared to 95 – 84 = 11 expected).

Table 12.1 (a) Estimate of the mean sojourn time (MST) and sensitivity in the Florence City Programme (age 50–69), based on interval and prevalence screening cancers. (b) Estimate of the mean sojourn time (MST) and sensitivity in the Florence City Programme (age 50–69), based on interval and incidence screening cancers

(a)	With TiS	Without TiS
MST (95% CI)	3.71 (3.25, 4.80)	3.42 (2.95, 4.08)
S (95% CI)	0.94 (0.79, 0.98)	0.95 (0.84, 0.98)

(b)	With TiS	Without TiS
MST (95% CI)	3.75 (2.52, 5.83)	3.98 (2.39, 7.70)
S (95% CI)	0.94 (0.81, 0.98)	0.96 (0.81, 0.98)

In the subsequent analysis the 'unbiased set' approach was used, excluding the breast cancer cases diagnosed at the prevalence screen. There were 51 interval cancer cases in the 2.42 years average interval and 89 screen-detected breast cancer cases at the incidence screen. Since 29 161 women attended the first screening test and 28 926 were screened negative, but only 21 504 attended the second, we estimated the person-years at risk (PY) in the interval, weighting for the contribution of each diagnostic modality (interval or screen-detection) to the total number of cases. This gave the number of person-years of $2.42 \times (28\ 926 \times 51/140 + 21\ 504 \times 89/140) = 58\ 502$.

The number of PY was also estimated including women not attending, to estimate the impact on the invited population. The PY denominator was estimated as before but adding breast cancer cases occurring in non-respondents:

$$PY = 2.42 \times (53\ 579 - 235) \times 162/251 + 21\ 504 \times 89/251 = 101\ 613$$

The ratio of the total incidence rate in the 'unbiased set' plus the non-respondents compared to the incidence in NYI women was:

$$RR = \frac{251/101\ 631}{284/116\ 715} = 1.01$$

with 95% confidence interval (0.85–1.20).

The expected number of incident cases in women responding to the invitation (unbiased set, PY = 58 502), after correction for the incidence rate in non-responders, was 136.3 versus the 140 cases observed (O/E ratio = 1.03)

Table 12.2 shows the stage distribution in the invited and NYI groups, with the predicted deaths. Table 12.3 gives the corresponding figures for the unbiased set and their expected values from the NYI group corrected for non-responders. Table 12.4 shows the stage distribution and predicted deaths for the non-responders alone. The invited population showed a small reduction of stage II+ breast cancer cases:

$$RR = \frac{114/101\ 631}{145/116\ 715} = 0.90$$

with 95% confidence interval (0.70, 1.16).

To assess the changing burden of the advanced carcinomas in the unbiased set only, we take into account that the occurrence of stage II+ breast cancer cases in the NYI group was lower than that in non-respondents. The stage II+ incidence rates were 1.24/1000 PY

Table 12.2 Predicted deaths in the invited population vs the NYI population

Stage	Invited women		NYI women	
	Number of cases	Number of predicted deaths	Number of cases	Number of predicted deaths
0–1	125	8.91	121	8.63
II+	114	47.38	145	60.26
NK	12	3.86	18	5.78
Total predicted deaths		59.34		74.67

Table 12.3 Predicted deaths in the unbiased set and expected numbers from the corrected NYI

Stage	Unbiased set observed cases	Unbiased set observed cases number of predicted deaths	Expected cases	Expected number of predicted deaths
0–1	84	5.96	64.93	4.63
II+	51	21.23	63.18	26.26
NK	5	1.60	8.19	2.63
Total predicted deaths	140	28.79	136.30	33.52

Table 12.4 Predicted deaths in non-responders

Stage	Non-responders number of cases	Non-responders number of predicted deaths
0–1	41	2.92
II+	63	29.36
NK	7	2.24
Total predicted deaths		34.52

in the NYI and 1.46/1000 PY in non-respondent women. As described above, the stage II+ expected incidence rate in the responders is estimated as 1.08/1000 PY and the observed to expected ratio is 51/63.10 = 0.81, with approximate 95% confidence interval (0.56, 1.18), a reduction in advanced stage tumours of 19%.

The relative risk of predicted death from breast cancer at 10 years for the invited group relative to the NYI, is calculated from Table 12.2 as

$$RR = \frac{59.34/101\,631}{74.67/116\,715} = 0.91$$

with 95% confidence interval (0.74–1.12). Comparing the unbiased set predicted deaths of 28.79 with those expected from the corrected NYI rates of 33.52 (Table 12.3), we obtain a relative risk of 0.86 with a 95% confidence interval of (0.64, 1.16).

12.6 Discussion

The above demonstrates simple methods for checking for over-diagnosis and predicting the mortality benefit in a breast cancer screening programme. We found no evidence of over-diagnosis in the Florence programme. The incidence of breast cancer in the Florence population is shown in Figure 12.2, with the percentage screen-detected. The observed increase in incidence as screening was introduced is consistent with cases being anticipated by lead time in screening, since the number of cases is as predicted by the sensitivity of screening and the mean sojourn time. The major conclusion of the early evaluation of the

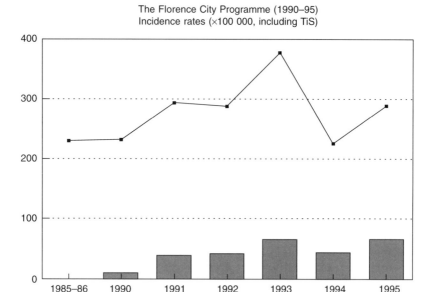

Figure 12.2 Incidence of breast cancer and percentage of cases screen detected by time in Florence

Florence breast cancer screening programme is that a population-based, high-quality screening programme can achieve a modest reduction in advanced cases and a subsequent reduction in mortality without a substantial increase in the number of diagnosed breast cancer cases. Furthermore, our data suggest that the occurrence of *in situ* carcinomas increased as a consequence of the screening programme but at the same time the number of invasive carcinomas decreased, compared with the expected numbers in the absence of screening. This suggests that some of the benefit of screening may be from a shift from invasive to carcinoma *in situ*, although the major benefit is a reduction in stage of invasive tumours.

We arrived at these conclusions in three steps:

1. The numbers of breast cancer cases at the prevalence and incidence screens were very well predicted from the estimates of the MST and *S*, suggesting that over-diagnosis was not present in the programme at the initial or at the subsequent screening test.
2. The use of the subset of data defined as the 'unbiased set' allowed for the comparison of the observed with the expected data excluding cases which might be affected by length bias.
3. Given the very similar number of cases in the two comparable populations the shift of stage towards *in situ* carcinomas and, in general, the decreasing rate of advanced carcinomas suggest that screening is starting to show an impact in terms of improving the stage distribution. The effect can be expressed as predicted deaths.

The programme has been running only a short time, and there is still considerable uncertainty about the benefit, as shown by the wide confidence intervals around the relative risk estimates. In future years, a more precise prediction of mortality reduction will be possible. Nevertheless there is a trend towards a reduction in incidence of advanced carcinoma, and the reduction is expected to be more evident in future.

The analysis we have presented in this paper confirms that the process of screening is apparently as expected, bearing in mind that further observation will enable more precise estimation. Also, considering a more detailed classification of tumour size and node status as simply stage I or stage II+, and including malignancy grade, will allow better estimation of the likely mortality reduction. The compliance rate of the target population is a major determinant of the impact of screening on the whole target population and the result observed in the Florence programme is heavily influenced by the low participation rate.

References

Day, N.E. and Duffy, S.W. (1996). Trial design based on surrogate endpoints: application to comparison of different breast screening frequencies. *Journal of the Royal Statistical Society A*, **159**, 49–60.

Day, N.E., Williams, D.D.R. and Khaw, K. (1989). Breast cancer screening programmes: the development of a monitoring and evaluation system. *British Journal of Cancer*, **59**, 954–8.

Day, N.E., McCann, J., Camilleri-Ferrante, C., Britton, P., Hurst, G., Cush, S. and Duffy, S.W. (1995). Monitoring interval cancers in breast screening programmes: the East Anglian experience. *Journal of Medical Screening*, **2**, 180–5.

Ernster, V.L. and Barclay, J. (1997). Increases in ductal carcinoma *in situ* (DCIS) of the breast in relation to mammography: a dilemma. *Monographs of the National Cancer Institute*, **22**, 151–6.

Moss, S.M., Michel, M., Patnick, J., Johns, L., Blanks, R. and Chamberlain, J. (1995). Results from the NHS breast screening programme 1990–1993. *Journal of Medical Screening*, **2**, 186–90.

Organizing Committee and Collaborators, Falun Meeting (1996). Breast cancer screening with mammography in women aged 40–49 years. *International Journal of Cancer*, **68**, 693–9.

Prevost, T.C., Launoy, G., Duffy, S.W. and Chen, H.H. (1998). Estimating sensitivity and sojourn time in screening for colorectal cancer – a comparison of statistical approaches. *American Journal of Epidemiology*, **133**, 832–8.

Tabar, L. (1995). Breast screening in Britain (editorial). *Journal of Medical Screening*, **2**, 179.

Tabar, L., Fagerberg, G., Chen, H.H., Duffy, S.W., Smart, C.R., Gad, A. and Smith, R.A. (1995). Efficacy of breast cancer screening by age: new results from the Swedish Two-County Trial. *Cancer*, **75**, 2507–17.

UICC (1987). *TNM Classification of Malignant Tumours*. International Union Against Cancer, Geneva.

van Ineveld, B.M., van Oortmarssen, G.J., de Koning, H.J., Boer, R. and van der Maas, P.J. (1993). How cost-effective is breast cancer screening in different EC countries? *European Journal of Cancer*, **12**, 1663–8.

13

Assessment of a colorectal cancer screening programme taking account of the natural history of the disease

Guy Launoy and Teresa C. Prevost

13.1 Introduction

The primary objective of cancer screening is to detect the disease as early as possible, or even as a precancerous lesion, so that treatment reduces the risk of dying from the disease. The characteristics of the natural history of the disease have therefore strong influences on the potential benefit of screening for that disease. Cancer screening is generally carried out on asymptomatic subjects, and its efficacy will depend on the period, called the sojourn time, when the person is asymptomatic but the disease is detectable by a screening tool. For a given cancer, the sojourn time varies between persons depending on pathologic and host factors. The parameter estimated in practice in screening programmes is the average sojourn time over all disease cases, usually referred to as the mean sojourn time (MST).

The longer the MST, the greater the potential advance in diagnosis from screening, and thus the expected long-term benefit of screening. The shorter the MST, the more frequently screening has to take place to have a chance of detecting the disease before symptoms. At the extreme, if the MST is very short, screening may not be worthwhile at all. The duration of preclinical disease is unknown for the majority of cancers. Extensive work has been done on quantitative theories of carcinogenesis, entailing numerous biological assumptions (Albert *et al.*, 1978; Thompson and Brown, 1987; Stevenson, 1995). The data provided by screening programmes represent the best opportunity to assess the duration of the preclinical time of a disease. Therefore, a considerable body of literature has been built up on the estimation of MST using screening-derived data (Day and Walter, 1984; van Oortmarssen *et al.*, 1990; Duffy *et al.*, 1995; Stevenson, 1995).

A second crucial element determining the efficacy of screening is the sensitivity of the test. The sensitivity of the test must be distinguished from the sensitivity of the programme although their estimations are usually confused. The test sensitivity is defined as the probability that a cancer in the preclinical detectable phase at a given time will be detected as positive if the screening test is applied at that time. The programme sensitivity is the proportion of cancers which will be screen-detected during a screening programme. Clearly the latter is dependent on the test sensitivity, the MST and the interval between screens. The sensitivity of the programme can be estimated approximately by $a/(a + c)$ where a is the number of cancers picked up by screening and c the number of cancers occurring clinically in the programme during a given period after the test. A better estimate of programme sensitivity uses the same formula, but defines a as the number of cancers detected at the nth screen (where n is at least 2) and c the cancers arising clinically between the $(n - 1)$th and the nth screen (see Chapter 8). As demonstrated by Day (1985), this ratio is not a valid estimator of the test sensitivity because it neglects the temporal aspect of cancer screening. The number c can include cases not yet in the preclinical screen-detectable phase at the time of the test, and it omits cases missed at the screening which do not become symptomatic before the next screen. Clearly, the number of tumours in these categories depends on the MST as well as the sensitivity of the test. To be reliable, therefore, an estimate of test sensitivity derived from screening data has to take into account the natural history of the cancer, in particular the MST.

Due to the frequency of colorectal cancer, and to the serious nature of the disease, screening for colorectal cancer is a major issue for public health in many industrialised countries. The efficacy of screening by the regular use of the faecal occult blood test (FOBT) has been established in three randomised trials which have each yielded a significant reduction in mortality from colorectal cancer using this test (Mandel et al., 1993; Hardcastle et al., 1996; Kronborg et al., 1996). It should be noted, however, that in one trial (Mandel et al., 1993) a high proportion of subjects underwent sigmoidoscopy, and that results varied by interval between screens. Reliable estimation of MST and sensitivity of the test are thus of interest in terms of explaining the variation in results already observed and of predicting the likely outcomes of alternative screening strategies.

The problem of estimating test sensitivity and MST using available data from screening programmes has received considerable attention in the last 20 years, and a range of modelling techniques is now available (Stevenson, 1995). Probably because of the availability of extensive data from randomised trials, most of the models have been applied to breast cancer screening, and relatively few to screening for colorectal cancer (Shapiro et al., 1974; Walter and Day, 1983; Day and Walter, 1984; Duffy et al., 1995; Paci and Duffy, 1991).

The aim of this study was to provide reliable estimates of sensitivity of FOBT which take into account the natural history of the disease. The strategy was to estimate the mean sojourn time and sensitivity together, so that each parameter was estimated taking the other into account. Moreover, since clinical, epidemiological and genetic evidence together suggest differences in natural history according to the tumour's location within the large bowel (Ponz de Leon et al., 1990; Buffil, 1991; Inoue et al., 1995), MST and test sensitivity were estimated separately for proximal colon, distal colon and rectum. Using these estimates, we investigated the influence of the interval between two screening tests on the sensitivity of the screening programme.

13.2 Screening data available

A first round of mass screening for colorectal cancer using FOBT was conducted in the French department of Calvados between April 1991 and May 1994. 164 634 people aged 45–74 years were invited for screening. The participation rate was 39% in males (30 215/77 049) and 47% in females (41 092/87 315). Test rehydration was not performed. There were a total of 1986 (2.8%) positive tests. Colonoscopy was performed in 816 males and 787 females, yielding respectively 81 and 50 cancers (Launoy *et al.*, 1996). For a three-year period following the test achievement, any cancer occurring in the negatively screened subjects was recorded, with the number of person-years of follow-up. Follow-up after the screening test ranged from 18 to 73 months. The number of tumours by sex, age at detection and location are shown in Table 13.1.

Table 13.1 Numbers of screen-detected and interval cancers by age and subsite*

Age	Detection mode	Proximal colon	Distal colon	Rectum	Unknown	All sites	Number of positive tests	Number screened
45–54							496	25 041
	Screened	3	7	2	0	12		
	Interval cancer	1	3	5	0	9		
55–64							722	24 933
	Screened	5	22	7	1	35		
	Interval cancer	8	12	10	1	31		
65–74							768	19 836
	Screened	17	51	15	1	84		
	Interval cancer	12	24	16	3	55		
45–74							1986	69 810
	Screened	25	80	24	2	131		
	Interval cancer	21	39	31	4	95		

*1497 attendants with unknown age were excluded

13.3 Statistical methods

A first empirical approach can be developed by comparing numbers of cancers in the attendant group with the expected numbers in the absence of screening. The latter was estimated using incidence rates provided by the Cancer Registry in the same area for the period 1978–90, i.e. just before screening started. All comparisons were adjusted for sex and age, using standardisation based on the general population of Calvados. The observed number of cases detected at screening (P) was compared with the number of expected incident cases in one year in the absence of screening (E_P) for each cancer location. For given sex and age, P/E_P depends on the MST and the test sensitivity: the longer the MST, the higher the P/E_P and the higher the sensitivity, the higher the P/E_P. If sensitivity is 100%, P/E_P is an estimate of the MST.

Similarly, the observed number of cases occurring after a negative test (N) was compared with the number of expected cases for the three-year period after the test (E_N). Let N_1, N_2 and N_3 be the number of cases occurring during the first, the second and the third year after the test respectively, and N_a be the total number. The corresponding expected numbers in the absence of screening are denoted by $E_{N_1}, E_{N_2}, E_{N_3}$ and E_{N_a}. The higher the sensitivity, the fewer post-screening cases will arise and therefore the lower will be N_a/E_{N_a}. The ratio N_1/E_{N_1} is in principle influenced more by sensitivity than the corresponding ratios in following years. One would expect N/E_N to increase towards unity, in successive years, at a rate inversely dependent on the MST. That is, the longer the time since last screen, the closer the clinical cancer incidence will be to the incidence in the absence of screening.

Finally, the observed number of cases occurring in the whole attendant group (A) was compared with the number of expected cases (E_A) for the three-year period after the test. The various ratios were estimated for each cancer location: proximal colon cancer (including caecum, ascending colon, transverse colon and splenic flexure), distal colon cancer (including descending colon, sigmoid colon and rectosigmoid junction) and rectal cancer (including rectal ampulla).

As a second approach, we modelled the incidence of cancers occurring after a negative test as a function of the sensitivity of the test and the MST. An exponential distribution with parameter λ is assumed for the duration of the sojourn time, thereby implying that the transition rate from preclinical disease to clinical disease is constant over time. Prevost *et al.* (1998) show that the incidence of cancers not existing at the time of the test and surfacing t years after the test can be approximated by:

$$I(t, \lambda) = I_e(1 - e^{-\lambda t})$$

where I_e is the incidence expected in the absence of screening.

When clinical disease occurs t years after screening in a person incorrectly screened as negative, this means that preclinical disease was present at the time of screening and the duration of the preclinical screen-detectable period was at least t years. Thus, incidence of cancers missed by the test and arising t years after the screening ($t = 0.5, 1.5, 2.5, \ldots$ representing the periods 0–1, 1–2, 2–3 years, and so on) can be estimated by:

$$J(t, \lambda, S_t) = a((1 - S_t)/S_t) \, [e^{-\lambda(t-0.5)} - e^{-\lambda(t+0.5)}]$$

Finally, the total incidence of cancers occurring after a negative test can be estimated as the sum of the above two quantities:

$$I(t, \lambda, S_t) = I(t, \lambda) + J(t, \lambda, S_t)$$

Several approaches can be used for parameter estimation (Prevost *et al.*, 1998). Here we present the estimates using Gibbs sampling for estimation (Gelfand and Smith, 1990). In this Bayesian approach, using the joint probability distribution for the unknown parameters, values from the marginal posterior distributions of the relevant parameters are repeatedly sampled from (Gibbs sampling) until approximate convergence to the unconditional posterior distributions. The method is implemented by the BUGS software, and the programming codes for these models are given by Prevost *et al.* (1998). From the sampled values obtained after convergence, empirical estimates of summary statistics for the parameters of interest are calculated. The method requires specification of prior distributions for the parameters. We used essentially flat priors to give results corresponding to a classical likelihood analysis. Results are given stratified first by age, and second by location.

Assuming an exponential distribution of the MST, λ as the parameter, we used the estimates of test sensitivity and mean sojourn time to predict potential programme sensitivity using the formula derived by Launoy *et al.* (1998):

$$S_p = \frac{S_t}{\lambda r}(1 - e^{-\lambda r}) \cdot \frac{1}{1 - ((1 - S_t)\,e^{-\lambda r})}$$

with *r* being the interval between two screening tests.

13.4 Results

13.4.1 First empirical approach

The first three columns of Table 13.2 show the screen-detected cancers and the ratio of these (P/E_P) to the expected incidence in the screened population in one year in the absence of screening. The ratio varied considerably by subsite for both sexes, being higher for distal colon in comparison with rectum or with proximal colon. This suggests that either MST, or sensitivity, or both were highest for distal colon cancer and lowest for

Table 13.2 Observed and expected* numbers of cases of colorectal cancer according to subsite in positive tests, negative tests and all attendants

	Positive tests			Negative tests			All attendants		
	OBS (*P*)	EXP (E_P)	P/E_P	OBS (*N*)	EXP (E_N)	N/E_N	OBS (*A*)	EXP (E_A)	A/E_A
Males									
Proximal	15	4.7	3.2	8	13.6	0.6	23	14.2	1.6
Distal	50	11.3	4.4	21	32.7	0.6	71	34.1	2.1
Rectum	14	9.0	1.6	19	26.0	0.7	33	27.0	1.2
Unknown	2	0.5	4.0	3	1.5	2.0	5	1.5	3.3
All sites	81	25.6	3.2	51	73.8	0.7	132	76.8	1.7
Females									
Proximal	10	6.0	1.7	13	17.5	0.7	23	18.0	1.3
Distal	30	9.9	3.0	18	29.0	0.6	48	29.8	1.6
Rectum	10	6.4	1.6	12	18.6	0.7	22	19.1	1.2
Unknown	0	0.7	0	1	2.0	0.5	1	2.0	0.5
All sites	50	23.0	2.2	44	67.1	0.7	94	68.9	1.4
Both sexes									
Proximal	25	10.7	2.3	21	31.1	0.7	46	32.2	1.4
Distal	80	21.3	3.8	39	61.8	0.6	119	63.8	1.9
Rectum	24	15.4	1.6	31	44.6	0.7	55	46.1	1.2
Unknown	2	1.2	1.7	4	3.5	1.1	6	3.5	1.7
All sites	131	48.5	2.7	95	141.0	0.7	226	145.6	1.6

*Age-standardised expected number of cases (in one year for positive tests, in three years for negative tests and all attendants) in the absence of screening, using 1978–1990 Calvados digestive cancer registry data

cancer of the rectum. Assuming a sensitivity of 100%, we would have estimated MSTs of 2–3 years for cancers of the proximal colon, 3–4 years for distal colon and 1–2 years for rectum.

The fourth-to-sixth columns of the table show the interval cancers, those expected in the absence of screening in three years (the average follow-up time) in a population the size of that screened negative, and the ratio of the two which is the proportional interval cancer incidence. The proportional interval cancer incidence estimates (N/E_N) for each subsite were very close to each other (0.6–0.7 for both sexes and all locations), suggesting that sensitivity did not vary substantially by subsite, and was only slightly lower for distal colon cancer and higher for proximal cancer.

On the whole, this approach suggested important variations in mean sojourn time according to cancer subsite, distal colon cancer presenting the longest MST (highest P/E_P) and rectal cancer the shortest (lowest P/E_P), with sensitivity not varying substantially. These results are, however, marginal in that the estimates of MST do not take sensitivity into account and the informal assessment of sensitivity from interval cancer incidence does not take sojourn time into account.

13.4.2 Modelling results on MST and sensitivity adjusted for each other

Table 13.3 shows the estimates of MST and sensitivity adjusted for each other, and stratified by age and location. Overall, the MST was estimated as 4.7 years and increased with age, three times longer for the oldest group (6.71 years) in comparison with the youngest (2.05). The MST was much higher for distal colon cancer (6.44) than others, that of proximal colon cancer (3.49) slightly higher than that of rectal cancer (2.61). Test sensitivity was estimated to be about 50%, twice as high in the youngest group (80%) in comparison with the oldest (40%). Test sensitivity did not vary substantially according to location, being only slightly higher for proximal cancer. The goodness of fit for the model was the best for proximal colon cancer and worst for distal colon cancer.

Comparing these results with those in Table 13.2, the inference is that the overall prevalence of 2.7 years of incidence masks a sojourn time of close to twice that figure (4.7) but a sensitivity of around 50%. The difference is most clearly seen for distal colon

Table 13.3 Estimates of mean sojourn time (MST) and sensitivity by age and location

	MST (CI)	Sensitivity (CI)
Age		
45–54 years	2.05 (1.00–12.50)	0.80 (0.18–0.98)
55–64 years	3.34 (1.49–12.50)	0.52 (0.17–0.91)
65–74 years	6.71 (3.70–16.73)	0.40 (0.18–0.63)
Location		
Proximal colon	3.49 (1.62–11.26)	0.55 (0.21–0.91)
Distal colon	6.44 (3.87–14.75)	0.49 (0.25–0.70)
Rectum	2.61 (1.15–11.20)	0.50 (0.15–0.88)
All	4.70 (3.06–8.35)	0.48 (0.30–0.66)

cancer. This demonstrates that the naive estimation of MST by the prevalence-to-incidence ratio can be unreliable if sensitivity is relatively poor.

13.4.3 Predicting the sensitivity of a programme

Table 13.4 shows the prediction for the sensitivity of the programme according to test sensitivity and screening frequency applying the formula given above for S_p for each location. Regarding all locations, for a given screening frequency, an increase of 10% in the test sensitivity provides a gain of 6% for the programme sensitivity. For a given test sensitivity, a gain of about 10% is obtained by switching from a triennial to a biennial screening regime, and about 15% from biennial to annual screening. It is notable that the model applies whether or not the screening frequency is shorter than the mean sojourn time.

13.5   Limitations, alternatives and implications

The great majority of available estimations of FOBT sensitivity have been calculated using the ratio $a/(a + c)$ where a is the number of cancers picked up by screening and c the number of cancers occurring during a given period (usually 1–2 years) after the test. This includes as false negatives those cancers which were not yet in the preclinical detectable phase at the time of the screen but which surfaced as clinical cancers within one year, and excludes those missed at the screen which reach the clinical phase after one year. These estimates obviously depend on the duration of follow-up after screening. With a one-year follow-up, sensitivity (after rehydration of the test) was estimated to be

Table 13.4 Sensitivity of the programme for each cancer location according to test sensitivity (S_t) and screening frequency (R) (MST = mean sojourn time)

	$r = 1$	$r = 2$	$r = 3$
$S_t = 40\%$			
Proximal colon (MST = 3.49)	0.62	0.46	0.36
Distal colon (MST = 6.44)	0.76	0.60	0.50
Rectum (MST = 2.61)	0.57	0.39	0.30
All locations (MST = 4.70)	0.70	0.54	0.44
$S_t = 50\%$			
Proximal colon (MST = 3.49)	0.69	0.53	0.43
Distal colon (MST = 6.44)	0.82	0.66	0.61
Rectum (MST = 2.61)	0.64	0.46	0.36
All locations (MST = 4.70)	0.76	0.60	0.50
$S_t = 60\%$			
Proximal colon (MST = 3.49)	0.74	0.59	0.48
Distal colon (MST = 6.44)	0.86	0.80	0.75
Rectum (MST = 2.61)	0.69	0.52	0.41
All locations (MST = 4.70)	0.80	0.66	0.56

80% (Mandel *et al.*, 1989, 1993). With a two-year follow-up, which is more generally chosen, estimates range from 37% to 68% (Allison *et al.*, 1996; Robinson *et al.*, 1995; Thomas *et al.*, 1992), rehydration of tests carrying a higher sensitivity (Mandel *et al.*, 1989; Kewenter *et al.*, 1994).

Using the above ratio estimate, our data would provide a sensitivity of 64% after one year and 58% after two years. In fact, since MST was estimated as between 4.5 and 5 years, the time spent in the preclinical phase of disease is expected to be sufficiently high that a follow-up of two years will accumulate less than half of the cancers missed by the test, and in this way, these estimates are likely to over-estimate the true sensitivity. On the other hand, the proportion of cases not existing at the time of the test out of the number of cancers occurring within two years after the test is unknown. Consideration of sensitivity without MST, or vice versa, is clearly unreliable. Taking into account the natural history is strongly suggested, to obtain reliable estimates of test sensitivity.

Our method has its own limitations. Firstly the assumption of a constant sensitivity and a variable sojourn time may itself be a simplification. There may be a sensitivity which begins at zero and increases as the tumour grows (at a varying rate from one case to another). This would be difficult to model, and our results suggest that an exponentially distributed sojourn time at a constant sensitivity gives a reasonable fit to our data, if MST and sensitivity are estimated simultaneously.

Three other phenomena are not taken into account by the method: firstly, the possibility of over-diagnosis at the prevalence screen is neglected. Secondly, due to the heightened awareness of the disease and its symptoms which might be expected during the screening campaign, a proportion of the interval cancers may also be diagnosed in advance of the time of diagnosis expected in the absence of a screening programme. This is all the more important since our analysis is based on one round of screening only. Conversely, the opposite phenomenon of delay in seeking medical attention for symptoms may occur in those reassured by a recent negative screen.

Others have obtained rather different estimates, notably of MST. The study in Fünen county, Denmark, gave estimates of test sensitivity of 56–62% and mean sojourn times of 2.21–2.78 years (Gyrd-Hansen *et al.*, 1997). These differences may be partly explained by differences in the age and sex distributions of attendants between the Fünen study population and our own.

Concerning the relationship between sensitivity of the programme and sensitivity of the screening test, Church *et al.* (1997) have recently suggested an alternative approach as follows:

$$S_p = 1 - \prod_{i=1}^{k} (1 - S(t_i))$$

for a cancer with a preclinical duration of k screens, with $S(t_i)$ being the screen sensitivity for the time t_i in the disease's development. As the authors indicate, this formula is relevant only if the cancers having a preclinical duration longer than the interval between two screens represent the vast majority of cases.

With regard to analysis by location, estimates of MST and test sensitivity from the Gibbs sampling method are consistent in qualitative terms with the first empirical approach. As a whole, our results strongly suggest that tumour progression rates were very different according to location, slowest for distal cancer and fastest for rectal cancer. This is also consistent with several studies which indicate underlying differences in clinical, epidemiological and genetic characteristics of cancers of the proximal colon, distal colon and rectum (Buffil, 1991; Inoue *et al.*, 1995; Ponz de Leon *et al.*, 1990). Regarding sensitivity and location, conclusions are very different depending on whether or not sensitivity is estimated taking account of MST. Ignoring MST, the test sensitivity appears to be lowest for cancer of the rectum and highest for distal colon (Thomas *et al.*, 1992). On the other hand, when MST was taken into account, sensitivity estimates for different locations were very close to each other, with a slightly higher value for proximal colon cancer. This surface discrepancy is completely explained by the variation in MST. Distal colon cancer having by far the longest MST, the over-estimation of actual sensitivity ignoring MST was greater for this location.

We have presented results estimated using the Bayesian technique of Gibbs sampling, as this is particularly convenient for complex models. It should be noted, however, that similar results were obtained using maximum likelihood estimation (Prevost *et al.*, 1998).

Two implications for screening practice are suggested by this study. Firstly, the low sensitivity of the Haemoccult test should stimulate research on other screening tests, such as the immunological faecal occult blood test, which is expected to be more sensitive than the chemical test which is mainly used currently (Castiglione *et al.*, 1994; Allison *et al.*, 1996; Robinson *et al.*, 1996; Nakama *et al.*, 1996). Secondly, the fact that the FOBT sensitivity was similarly poor for distal colon and rectal cancer suggests that combining FOBT and sigmoidoscopy could be a good strategy for colorectal cancer screening, as suggested by the Danish randomised study findings (Kronborg *et al.*, 1996).

In terms of evaluation, the major implication is that evaluation of disease screening programmes can be assisted by taking into account features of the disease process. In particular, sensitivity should be estimated taking into account the time the disease spends in the preclinical screen-detectable phase.

References

Albert, A., Gertman, P.M. and Louis, T.A. (1978). Screening for the early detection of cancer. I. The temporal natural history of a progressive disease state. *Mathematic Bioscience*, **40**, 1–59.

Allison, J.E., Tekawa, I.S., Ransom, L.J. and Adrain, A.L. (1996). A comparison of faecal occult-blood tests for colorectal cancer screening. *N. Engl. J. Med.*, **334**,155–9.

Buffil, J.A. (1991). Colorectal cancer, evidence for distinct genetic categories based on proximal or distal tumor location. *Ann. Intern. Med.*, **114**, 431–2.

Castiglione, G., Sala, P., Ciatto, S., Grazzini, G., Mazzotta, A., Rossetti, C., Spinelli, P. and Bertario, L. (1994). Comparative analysis of results of guaiac and immunochemical tests for faecal occult blood in colorectal cancer screening in two oncological institutions. *Eur. J. Cancer Prev.*, **3**, 399–405.

Church, T.R., Ederer, F. and Mandel, J.S. (1997). Fecal occult blood screening in the Minnesota study: sensitivity of the screening test. *J. Natl. Cancer Inst.*, **89**, 1440–8.

Day, N.E. (1985). Estimating the sensitivity of a screening test. *J. Epidemiol. Commun. Health*, **39**, 364–6.

Day, N.E. and Walter, S.D. (1984). Simplified models of screening for chronic disease, estimation procedures from mass screening programmes. *Biometrics*, **43**, 1–56.

Duffy, S.W., Chen, H.H., Tabar, L. and Day, N.E. (1995). Estimation of mean sojourn time in breast cancer screening using a Markov chain model of both entry to and exit from the preclinical detectable phase. *Stat. Med.*, **14**, 1531–44.

Gelfand, A.E. and Smith, A.F.M. (1990). Sampling based approaches to calculating marginal densities. *J. Am. Stat. Assoc.*, **85**, 398–409.

Gyrd-Hansen, D., Sogaard, J. and Kronborg, O. (1997). Analysis of screening data: colorectal cancer. *Int. J. Epidemiol.*, **26**, 1172–81.

Hardcastle, J.D., Chamberlain, J.O., Robinson, M.H. *et al.* (1996). Randomised controlled trial of faecal-occult-blood screening for colorectal cancer. *Lancet*, **348**, 1472–7.

Inoue, M., Tajima, K., Hirose, K. *et al.* (1995). Subsite-specific risk factors for colorectal cancer, a hospital-based case-control study in Japan. *Cancer Causes Control*, **6**, 14–22.

Kewenter, J., Brevinge, H., Engaras, B., Haglind, E. and Ahren, C. (1994). Results of screening, rescreening and follow-up in a prospective randomized study for detection of colorectal cancer by fecal occult blood testing. *Scand. J. Gastroenterol.*, **29**, 468–73.

Kronborg, O., Fenger, C., Olsen, J., Jorgensen, O.D. and Sondergaard, O. (1996). Randomised study of screening for colorectal cancer with faecal-occult-blood test. *Lancet*, **348**, 1467–71.

Launoy, G., Herbert, C., Vallee, J.P. *et al.* (1996). Le depistage de masse du cancer colorectal en France. Experience aupres de 165 000 personnes dans le Calvados, *Gastroenterol. Clin. Biol.*, **20**, 228–36.

Launoy, G., Duffy, S.W., Prevost, T.C. and Bouvier, V. (1998). Dépistage des cancers. Sensibilité du test et sensibilité du programme de dépistage. *Rev. Epidemiol. Santé Publ.*, **46**, 420–6.

Mandel, J.S., Bond, J.H., Bradley, M. *et al.* (1989). Sensitivity, specificity and positive predictivity of the Haemoccult test in screening for colorectal cancers. *Gastroenterology*, **97**, 597–600.

Mandel, J.S., Bond, J.H., Church, T.R. *et al.* (1993). Reducing mortality from colorectal cancer by screening for fecal occult blood. *N. Engl. J. Med.*, **328**, 1365–71.

Nakama, H., Kamijo, N., Fattah, A.S.M.A. and Zhang, B. (1996). Validity of immunological faecal occult blood screening for colorectal cancer, a follow-up study. *J. Med. Screening*, **3**, 63–5.

Paci, E. and Duffy, S.W. (1991). Modelling the analysis of breast cancer screening programmes: sensitivity, lead time and predictive value in the Florence district programme. *Int. J. Epidemiol.*, **20**, 852–8.

Ponz de Leon, M., Sacchetti, C., Sassatelli, R., Zanghieri, G., Roncucci, L. and Scalmati, A. (1990). Evidence for the existence of different types of large bowel tumor, suggestions from the clinical data of a population-based registry. *J. Surg. Oncol.*, **44**, 35–43.

Prevost, T.C., Launoy, G., Duffy, S.W. and Chen, H.H. (1998). Estimating sensitivity and sojourn time in screening for colorectal cancer: a comparison of statistical approaches. *Am. J. Epidemiol.*, **148**, 609–19.

Robinson, M.H.E., Moss, S.M., Hardcastle, J.D., Whynes, D.K., Chamberlain, J.O. and Mangham, C.M. (1995). Effect of retesting with dietary restriction in Haemoccult screening for colorectal cancer. *J. Med. Screening*, **2**, 41–4.

Robinson, M.H.E., Marks, C.G., Farrands, P.A., Bostock, K. and Hardcastle, J.D. (1996). Screening for colorectal cancer with an immunological faecal occult blood test: 2-year follow-up. *Br. J. Surg.*, **83**, 500–1.

Shapiro, S., Goldberg, J.D. and Hutchison, G.B. (1974). Lead time in breast cancer detection and implication for periodicity of screening. *Am. J. Epidemiol.*, **100**, 357–66.

Stevenson, C.E. (1995). Statistical models for cancer screening. *Stat. Methods Med. Research*, **4**, 18–32.

Thomas, W.M., Pye, G., Hardcastle, J.D. and Walker, A.R. (1992). Screening for colorectal carcinoma, an analysis of the sensitivity of Haemoccult. *Br. J. Surg.*, **79**, 833–5.

Thompson, J.R. and Brown, B.W. (1987). *Cancer Modelling*. Marcel Dekker, New York.

van Oortmarssen, G.J., Habbema, J.D., van der Maas, P.J., de Koning, H.J., Collette, H.J., Verbeek, A.L., Geerts, A.T. and Lubbe, K.T. (1990). A model for breast cancer screening. *Cancer*, **66**, 1601–12.

Walter, S.D. and Day, N.E. (1983). Estimation of the duration of a preclinical disease state using screening data. *Am. J. Epidemiol.*, **118**, 865–85.

14

Screening for neuroblastoma in children: insight gained from the modelling of various screening strategies

Jacques Estève, Stephen W. Duffy and Catherine Hill

14.1 Introduction

Neuroblastoma is a tumour of the sympathetic nervous system, which derives from embryonic cells of the neural crest. It occurs mainly in early childhood and is rare even in this age group. The incidence ranges from around 7 to 13 per million children in Europe but, according to unpublished data from the National Registry of Childhood Tumours, it accounts for 13% of cancer deaths in children in the UK (Powell *et al.*, 1997; Parkin *et al.*, 1998). In Europe, the risk of being diagnosed with neuroblastoma before 15 years of age is about $120/10^6$ and the risk of death from the disease $65/10^6$.

Since neuroblastoma occurs at various primary sites and since cancer registration is generally classified by site rather than histology (Mathieu *et al.*, 1993), its incidence and mortality cannot be assessed from routine Cancer Registry data. The above figures were obtained from *ad hoc* studies (Powell *et al.*, 1997; Parkin *et al.,* 1998), in which it may be seen that the incidence of the disease decreases rapidly with age, reaching a very low level after 5 years. Another striking aspect of the epidemiology of the disease is the contrasted survival probabilities between the children diagnosed before one year and after one year of age (Figure 14.1). Tumours diagnosed earlier in life have substantially better prognosis. Tumours presenting before one year tend to be at an early stage, but both age and stage are strong and independent predictors of survival (Evans *et al.*, 1987). These characteristics of the disease led clinicians to hypothesise that many neuroblastomas diagnosed after one year were already present without symptoms and at a more favourable stage for successful treatment at an earlier age. This in turn motivated a search for a method of detection of the disease at an early age, in a preclinical stage. Since it was

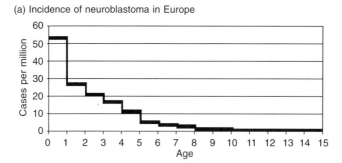

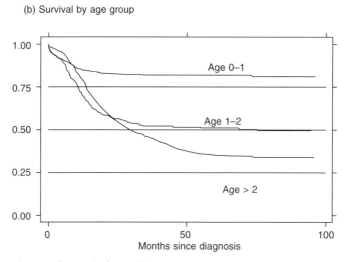

Figure 14.1 Incidence and survival of neuroblastoma by age

known that most tumours excreted abnormal levels of dopamine and of its metabolites, homovanillic acid (HVA) and vanillylmandelic acid (VMA), a simple non-invasive test was readily available if reliable measurement of these biochemical products could be made from urine samples. Various studies of screening in practice have been performed. The purpose of this article is to show that modelling the natural history of the disease can help screening study researchers to interpret their data, and can assist in designing more appropriate studies of screening efficacy than have been carried out to date.

The following sections will deal with the rationale for screening for neuroblastoma, a proposed model for disease progression, the expected prevalence of the disease at different ages and the consequent implications for mortality of screening at different ages, respectively. The work presented here is largely taken from previous work done within the Study Group for the Evaluation of Neuroblastoma Screening in Europe (*SENSE*) (Estève *et al.*, 1995, 1998; Erttmann *et al.*, 1998).

14.2 Rationale for neuroblastoma screening

In addition to the common belief that early diagnosis is always beneficial, there were several reasonable arguments to undertake screening for a rare disease such as neuroblastoma. The tumour was thought to be present at birth and had extremely good prognosis when diagnosed soon after it, but was much more likely to be fatal when diagnosed later, partly due to being more likely to be at a disseminated stage. No important therapeutic improvement was expected, and it was legitimate to try to find a method for detecting the tumour at or soon after birth, hoping that this would prevent its progression. The first mass screening of this type was implemented in the early 1980s in Japan (Sawada *et al.*, 1984, 1986) with no prior evaluation of its efficacy. Neuroblastoma screening was set up early after birth (3–6 months) with the expectation of a very large benefit, which was supported to some extent by the epidemiology of the disease (Figure 14.1). Several untested hypotheses are however implied by such a screening scheme:

1. Neuroblastoma is a tumour which is present at birth and which produces abnormal level of cathecolamine metabolites a long time before being symptomatic.
2. Neuroblastomas detected at screening due to excretion of high levels of HVA/VMA would have been diagnosed at a later age in the absence of screening.
3. All screen positive tumours will benefit from being detected early. In other words, the tumours so detected will have the same survival as the tumours presenting with symptoms before one year of age.

This reasoning was probably at the origin of the implementation of the Japanese programme that was set up in 1985 and thought to be successful, based on the excellent survival of the screen positive subjects. A non-randomised study aimed at evaluation of a programme screening for neuroblastoma at three weeks and six months was carried out in Quebec (Tuchmann *et al.,* 1990), but results are inconclusive, possibly due to the rather small study size for such a rare disorder (Estève *et al.*, 1995).

Some doubts about neuroblastoma screening were then expressed by the scientific community (Murphy *et al.,* 1991), and over a period of time over-diagnosis has been identified as the main drawback of the procedure (Carlsen, 1990, 1992; Goodman, 1991; Estève *et al.*, 1995). The establishment of over-diagnosis proved that hypothesis 2 above was wrong (although this does not in itself disprove efficacy of screening). If early screening were only detecting an almost benign disease or if the rare tumours with unfavourable genetic features detected at screening could not benefit from anticipating their diagnosis, there would be no room for a screening strategy in the control of the disease. Also, it is possible to imagine that screening later, between 12 and 18 months, could anticipate the diagnosis of the worse tumours while avoiding the detection of the benign tumours found at six months, which would have never surfaced in the absence of early screening.

This line of reasoning led us to try to model the natural history of the disease to estimate the benefit that could be expected from various screening strategies. The main idea was that early screening may detect the wrong tumours because the tumours with a bad prognosis do not excrete cathecolamine metabolites early enough. Since the benefit in mortality can only come from the detection of the potentially fatal tumours it is possible that later screening would produce a larger benefit.

14.3 The model

In the context of screening for neuroblastoma, the sojourn time, defined in Chapter 1, is

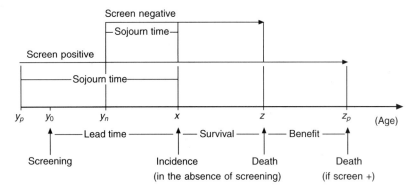

Figure 14.2 Diagram showing the main concepts of screening evaluation (see text)

the period within which the tumour excretes abnormal levels of HVA/VMA, and before it becomes clinically symptomatic. The cases which could benefit from screening are those which are in their sojourn time at the age at which a potential screening would take place. The number of such cases depends obviously on the incidence of the disease but more significantly on the length of the sojourn time. For example, when for a given case this time is shorter than the difference between age of incidence in the absence of screening and age at screening, the corresponding case will screen negative and no benefit is to be expected.

The potential benefit or lack of benefit is illustrated in Figure 14.2. Suppose y_0 is the age at screening, and consider those tumours which would become clinically symptomatic at age x, where $x > y_0$. Suppose also that in the absence of screening, such tumours would be expected to lead to death at age z. Now for screen-detected subjects, the survival is automatically increased by the *lead time*. Assume that in addition to this, the earlier stage at diagnosis due to screening confers an additional survival benefit, so that screen-detected subjects die at age $z_p > z$. Figure 14.2 shows the course of disease for two subjects, both of which would have been clinically detected at age x. For subject p (screen positive), the sojourn time begins (i.e. the tumour begins to excrete high levels of HVA/VMA) at age y_p before the screen at y_0. This subject will therefore be screened positive, have the diagnosis advanced to an earlier stage, and the death delayed to time z_p. For subject n (screen negative) the sojourn time begins at age y_n, after the screen at y_0. This subject will therefore be screened negative, will advance to clinical disease at age x and will die at age z.

Note that it is possible in principle that $z_p = z$ and the benefit is therefore zero. Also, the screening test may not be 100% sensitive, and so subject p may be missed at the test and therefore derive no benefit. In any case, the number of subjects who can benefit from screening is at most the number who are within their sojourn time at y_0, the age at screening.

In mathematical terms, if Y is the random variable defining the age at the start of the sojourn time, V the sojourn time itself and $f(x)$ the probability density of age at incidence (X), the probability that a case will be in the screen-detectable phase when screening takes place (y_0) is:

$$\text{Prob}(Y < y_0) = \int_{y_0}^{\infty} f(x)\,\text{Prob}(V > (x - y_0))\,dx$$

In other words the cases prevalent at screening are obtained from the sum, over all ages greater than y_0, of the cases which would occur clinically at age x in the absence of screening $f(x)$, and who would have a sojourn time sufficiently long ($\text{Prob}(V > (x - y_0))$). This latter term has to be estimated from a theoretical distribution reflecting present knowledge on the duration of this preclinical phase of the disease. Some clinical information, added to information on false negative cases in the various screening programmes (Berthold et al., 1991; Nakagawara et al., 1991; Ishimoto et al., 1990; Ertmann et al., 1998), suggested that the mean sojourn time was approximately 15 months. This information would be sufficient to model the sojourn distribution with an exponential density. Since, however, the sojourn time was constrained to be lower than age, it should have a lower mean and variance for early-age tumours. It was therefore considered more realistic to model sojourn time with a Weibull distribution:

$$\text{Prob}(V > v) = \exp[-(\mu v)^p]$$

where μ and p were chosen in such a way that the mean sojourn time varied from 16 months for a tumour occurring at age 2 years up to 19 months for tumours occurring at 5 years, while the standard deviation varied from 7.4 to 22 months in the same age interval (p was taken to change linearly with age and the distribution was truncated to meet the age constraint).

The integral above was approximated by a finite sum by subdivision of the age axis into three-month intervals in the first year, six-month intervals up to five years and one-year intervals up to 15 years. The function $f(x)$ was then evaluated at $(x_i + x_{i+1})/2$ as $\lambda_i(x_{i+1} - x_i)$, where λ_i is the proportional incidence, that is the incidence rate for age $(x_i + x_{i+1})/2$ divided by the total incidence rate to age 15, estimated from the limited registry data available from selected European countries.

14.4 Prevalence at screening

The above formula provides the proportion of *tumours* that are in their sojourn time at the time of screening. To return to the proportion of *children* who have a tumour in its preclinical phase at the time of screening (the prevalence at screening) we multiplied the result of the calculation of the integral by the estimated overall risk of neuroblastoma in Europe, 120 per million by age 15. Using this method it was shown that screening at 18 months would yield 29 cases per million children, screening at 12 months would yield 34.5 cases per million, and screening at six months would yield 40 cases per million. The last figure is well below the detection rates reported in Quebec (Woods et al., 1996) and Japan (Sawada et al., 1984). These were respectively 40 per million at three weeks followed by a further 74 per million at six months and 60 per million at six months. Since before screening, both populations had similar incidence rates to those from Europe used in our calculations, this demonstrates formally that in these two studies many cases detected by screening would not have become incident.

If we assume that the production of abnormal levels of metabolites is maintained

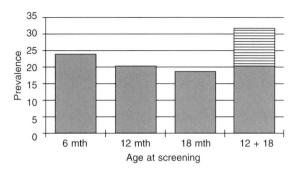

Figure 14.3 Prevalence (cases per million) with diagnosis anticipated by more than three months, by age at screening

uninterrupted after its inception, we can consider that the sensitivity of the test is 100% since an abnormal level has 100% chance of being detected by the procedures in use today (mainly high-performance liquid chromatography). In the following calculation we shall therefore consider that the prevalence at screening is also the detection rate.

Among the cases detected at screening, some have a very small lead time and would not benefit from it. We therefore assumed that no benefit was expected if the anticipation of diagnosis was less than three months. Based on the age-specific incidence and the distributions of sojourn times, it was calculated that among the cases prevalent at six months 24 could benefit from it, at 12 months 20.5, and at 18 months 19. These figures strongly suggest that the advantage of screening early should be minimal. In contrast, if screening were performed both at 12 and 18 months, a calculation along the same lines showed that a further 11.3 cases in addition to those benefiting from a screen at 12 months would have an anticipated diagnosis of at least three months. These results are summarised in Figure 14.3.

14.5 Effect of screening on mortality

As explained above, mortality figures for neuroblastoma are not routinely available except from some children's cancer registries or from *ad hoc* studies (Stiller, 1993). By combining incidence with survival, however, mortality can be calculated. Incidence rates from several national cancer registries were made available to us (Powell *et al.*, 1997) and survival figures are well known (see Figure 14.1). To calculate the reduction in mortality associated with a screening regime, we need estimates of the incidence by age and detection mode (screening or symptomatic) in a hypothetical screened population, and the expected survival probabilities in the screen-detected and symptomatic tumours. For symptomatic clinically detected tumours in the screened group (those reaching the end of the sojourn time before age at screening or moving into the sojourn time after the age at screening), the survival figures for an unscreened population were assumed. For screen-detected tumours, we postulated improved survival consistent with age-specific variation in survival illustrated in Figure 14.1, with the improvement increasing with increasing lead time (for example, a tumour whose diagnosis is advanced by one year derives a greater benefit than one whose diagnosis is advanced by six months). The hypothetical survival probabilities by lead time are shown in Table 14.1.

Table 14.1 Hypothetical survival probability (%) of screened detected cases by lead time achieved

Lead time (months)	Month since diagnosis			
	12	36	60	120
< 3		No benefit		
3–12	97	87	85	85
12–24	99	88	86	85
> 24	99	97	90	89

Table 14.2 and Figure 14.4 show the predicted effects on mortality of screening at different ages. The calculation of these figures is a relatively laborious procedure involving estimation of cases by age, detection mode and, where relevant, lead time, combined with survival probabilities relevant to these and for varying times from diagnosis to give the cumulative mortality specific to a given age. For example, tumours diagnosed at age three years need to have seven-year survival applied to calculate the cumulative mortality at 10 years. The basic principle, however, is illustrated in the following simple and very rough approximation for mortality to age 14 for an unscreened population and one screened at 12 months.

- One would expect around 120 cases per million up to age 14 (see Section 14.1).
- The vast majority of these will be diagnosed before age 5, so we need to estimate 10–14-year survival rates.
- From Figure 14.1, in an unscreened population, we would expect 54 per milllion incidents before age one year, 27 between first and second birthday and 39 from second birthday onwards.
- Also from Figure 14.1, we have survival to eight years. Assuming 10–14-year survival to be somewhat less than this, we might postulate 70% for tumours incident before age one, 40% for tumours incident between ages one and two, and 25% for tumours incident after age two.
- The total deaths in an unscreened group would then be 54 × 0.3 + 27 × 0.6 + 39 × 0.75 = 62 per million.
- For a population screened at 12 months one would expect 34 screen-detected cases

Table 14.2 Cumulative mortality from neuroblastoma according to various screening strategies

Screening strategy	Cumulative mortality at age[a] (years)					
	0	2	5	7	10	14
No screening	2.9	18.4	44.4	54.5	60.9	64.4
At 6 months	3.1	11.9	35.0	44.8	51.1	54.6
At 12 months	2.9	14.5	34.6	44.0	50.3	53.7
At 18 months	2.9	18.1	35.1	44.0	50.2	53.4
Both 12 and 18 months	2.9	14.5	29.2	37.7	43.8	47.0

[a]Cumulative risk of mortality up to the end of this year of age

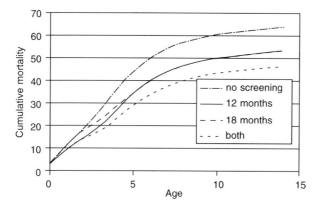

Figure 14.4 Mortality from neuroblastoma according to screening strategy

of which 21 will have a lead time of more than three months and will therefore benefit (see Section 14.4).

- We would expect these 21 cases to have a long-term survival of 85% (Table 14.1).
- Assume that 75% (16 cases) of the 21 anticipated cases who benefit are anticipated from the 1–2-year incidence and 25% (6 cases) from the incidence from two years of age onwards.
- The total deaths in a screened group would be $54 \times 0.3 + 21 \times 0.15 + 11 \times 0.6 + 34 \times 0.75 = 51$ per million.

It is interesting to note that the reduction in mortality is predicted to be of the order of 15% whatever the age at screening. It would reach 25% if screening were performed at both 12 and 18 months. As expected, postponing screening does not reduce efficacy but, given the hypothesis on sojourn time distribution, provides a negligible improvement. A smaller sojourn time would provide a larger improvement of late screening over early screening but would also reduce the overall efficacy of screening based on a once-only testing strategy.

The fact that the predicted mortality in the first year of life is slightly higher for screening at six months than for no screening at all may be thought of as the effect of ascertainment bias. The prevalence of screen detected tumours at six months combined with the theoretical, albeit low, fatality at six months gives a number of deaths higher than one would expect from no screening at all. This can happen in reality, since the identification of cases who would otherwise die undiagnosed artificially increases the mortality.

The estimated reduction demonstrates also that an efficacy trial would be extremely arduous to carry out. It can be calculated that it would be necessary to set up a programme in a population with one million births per year, test all the children during at least five years and follow them up five more years to have sufficient power (Estève *et al.*, 1995).

14.6 Discussion and conclusion

It is clear that the modelling of the natural history of neuroblastoma is approximate and would require more information on the excretion of cathecolamine metabolites. The postulated sojourn times, 14–20 months on average, during which tumours are excreting abnormal levels of VMA/HVA before being symptomatic are speculative, even if most tumours do so at diagnosis.

After publication of the Japanese results of an uncontrolled study of screening at six months, on 281 939 infants, there was a consensus for carrying out efficacy trials, including the geographically controlled study in Quebec (Tuchman *et al.*, 1990). The study designed in Quebec, with 476 603 children in the study group, and approximately one million infants in two control areas (Woods *et al.*, 1996) also under-estimated the number of subjects needed to confirm or refute the decrease in mortality that could be reasonably expected. In addition, the trial was not randomised. It might therefore be difficult to interpret the results of such a study, particularly in the context of the incidence increase that has been observed recently in several regions among infants. If, as suggested by a recent study (Powell *et al.*, 1997), early incidental diagnosis is the explanation for the incidence increase and if anticipation of diagnosis has some efficacy, a non-randomised comparison could be biased. The only acceptable approach, from a methodological point of view, would have been to analyse only a random half of the urine samples and to compare the mortality between the two arms so defined.

The most recent trial, also geographically controlled, undertaken in Germany (Schilling *et al.*, 1998) is planned to have 1 250 000 infants screened at 12 months in the study areas, and the same number not screened in the control areas. Although larger than the Japanese and Quebec studies it is still too small to demonstrate the efficacy of screening if the figures in Section 14.5 are correct, but it will at least yield useful information on over-diagnosis. The preliminary results suggest that postponing screening at this age is not enough to eliminate it.

The idea that the benefit could be less than that initially anticipated was reinforced by the molecular biology of the tumours (Brodeur *et al.*, 1998). Neuroblastomas detected by early screening were almost always near triploid in chromosome number or DNA content and lacked the genetic features associated with poor outcome (*MYC-N* amplification and chromosome 1p deletion). Thus, the biological evidence that is accumulating suggests that neuroblastoma is actually two diseases. One type acquires early the genetic features that are synonymous of very bad prognosis, and is unlikely to benefit from screening, and the other does not and so may benefit from screening (although this is by no means guaranteed).

The empirical evidence, from screening studies in the field, and from experimental laboratory observations on individual tumours, suggest exceptions to all three of the hypotheses listed in Section 14.2 which formed the basis of neuroblastoma screening. The first hypothesis that the tumour is present at birth and excretes cathecolamine metabolites long before symptoms is contradicted by the incidence of clinical tumours after a negative screen (Woods *et al.*, 1996). The second, that neuroblastomas detected at screening would have arisen naturally in the absence of screening, is inconsistent with the evidence of over-diagnosis and the almost uniformly favourable genetic features of screen-detected tumours. Both of the latter render the third hypothesis, that screen-detected tumours benefit in terms of survival, difficult to evaluate. The presence of over-diagnosis suggests that this is not universally true, and it is not possible to identify with any certainty those tumours which are over-diagnosed and those which would have arisen clinically and whose diagnosis has been advanced by the screening.

Despite its limitations, the modelling above for studying screening strategies for neuroblastoma achieved several goals. First, it confirmed that screening at six months generated heavy over-diagnosis and it gave some estimate of its size. Secondly, it showed that postponing screening would not reduce its efficacy. Third, it gave a quantitative estimate of the size of the reduction in mortality that could be expected from several screening strategies. It is clear that this effort should have been more relevant if it had been made before and not after screening programmes and efficacy trials were implemented.

Although there are some indications that a subgroup of neuroblastomas may benefit from an anticipated diagnosis (Powell *et al.*, 1997; Matsui *et al.*, 1994), the present consensus is rather against screening for neuroblastoma and even against undertaking any trial for testing its efficacy. The modelling reported in this chapter has partly contributed to this consensus.

References

Berthold, F., Hunneman, D.H., Käser, H., Harms, D., Bertram, U., Ertmann, R., Schilling, F.H., Treuner, J. and Zieschang, J. (1991). Neuroblastoma screening: arguments from retrospective analysis of three German neuroblastoma trials. *Am. J. Pediatr. Hematol. Oncol.*, **13**, 8–13.

Brodeur, G.M., Ambros, P.F. and Favrot, M.C. (1998). Biological aspects of neuroblastoma screening. *Med. Pediatr. Oncol.*, **31**, 394–400.

Carlsen, N.L.T. (1990). How frequent is spontaneous remission of neuroblastomas? Implications for screening. *Br. J. Cancer*, **61**, 441–6.

Carlsen, N.L.T. (1992). Neuroblastoma: epidemiology and pattern of regression. *Am. J. Pediat. Hematol. Oncol.*, **14**, 103–10.

Erttmann, R., Tafese, T., Berthold, F., Kerbl, R., Mann, J., Parker, L., Schilling, F., Ambros, P., Christiansen, H., Favrot, M., Kabisch, H., Hero, B. and Philip, T. on behalf of the SENSE group (1998). 10 years' neuroblastoma screening in Europe: preliminary results of a clinical and biological review from the study group for evaluation of neuroblastoma screening in Europe. *Eur. J. Cancer*, **34**, 1391–7.

Estève, J., Parker, L., Roy, P., Hermann, F., Duffy, S., Frappaz, D., Lasset, C., Hill, C., Sancho-Garnier, H., Michaelis, J. and Philip, T. (1995). Is neuroblastoma screening evaluation needed and feasible? *Br. J. Cancer*, **71**, 1125–31.

Estève, J., Roy, P., Chauvin, F. and Philip, T. (1998). Screening for neuroblastoma in children: elements for a statistical evaluation. *Am. Pediatr. Oncol.*, **31**, 401–7.

Evans, A.E., D'Angio, G.J., Propert, K., Anderson, J. and Hann, H.L. (1987). Prognostic factors in neuroblastoma. *Cancer*, **59**, 1853–9.

Goodman, S.N. (1991). Neuroblastoma screening data. An epidemiologic analysis. *Am. J. Dis. Child.*, **145**, 1415–22.

Ishimoto, K., Kiyokawa, N., Fujita, H., Yabuta, K., Ohya, T., Miyano, T. *et al.* (1990). Problems of mass screening for neuroblastoma: analysis of false-negative cases. *J. Pediat. Surg.*, **25**, 398–401.

Mathieu, P., Favrot, M., Frappaz, D., Chauvin, F., Greffe, J., Montegue, A. *et al.* (1993). Le neuroblastome de l'enfant: aspects cliniques et biologiques. Une expérience de dépistage en France. *Ann. Biol. Clin.*, **51**, 665–88.

Matsui, I., Tanimura, M., Kobayashi, N. *et al.* (1994). In: Sawada, T., Matsumura, T., Kizaki, Z. (eds). *Proceedings of the 3rd International Symposium on Neuroblastoma Screening*. Kyoto Prefectural University of Medicine, pp. 3–11.

Murphy, S.B., Cohn, S.L., Craft, A.W., Woods, W.G., Sawada, T., Castleberry, R.P. *et al.* (1991). Do children benefit from mass screening for neuroblastoma? *Lancet*, **337**, 344–6.

Nakagawara, A., Zaizen, Y., Ikeda, K., Ohgami, H., Nagahara, N., Sera, Y. *et al.* (1991). Different genomic and metabolic patterns between mass screening-positive and mass screening-negative later-presenting neuroblastomas. *Cancer*, **68**, 2037–44.

Parkin, D.M., Kramarova, E., Draper, G.J., Masuyer, E., Michaelis, J., Neglia, J., Qureshi, S. and Stiller, C.A. (eds) (1998). *International Incidence of Childhood Cancer, Vol. II*. International Agency for Research on Cancer, Lyon.

Powell, J.E., Estève, J., Mann, J.R., Parker, L., Frappaz, D., Michaelis, J. *et al.* (1997). Neuroblastoma in Europe: why is the pattern of disease different in Britain? *Lancet*, **352**, 682–7.

Sawada, T. (1986). Outcome of 25 neuroblastomas revealed by screening in Japan. *Lancet*, **i**, 377.

Sawada, T., Nakata, T., Takasugi, N., Maeda, K., Hanawa, Y., Shimizu, K. *et al.* (1984). Mass screening for neuroblastoma in infants in Japan. *Lancet*, **ii**, 271–3.

Schilling, F.H., Spix, C., Berthold, F., Erttmann, R., Hero, B., Michaelis, J., Sander, J., Tafese, T. and Treuner, J. (1998). German neuroblastoma mass screening study at 12 months of age: statistical aspects and preliminary results. *Med. Pediatr. Oncol.*, **31**, 435–41.

Stiller, C.A. (1993). Trends in neuroblastoma in Great Britain: incidence and mortality, 1971–1990. *Eur. J. Cancer*, **28A**, 1008–12.

Tuchman, M., Lemieux, B., Auray-Blais, C., Robison, L.L., Giguere, R., McCann, M.T. and Woods, W.G. (1990). Screening for neuroblastoma at 3 weeks of age: methods and preliminary results from the Quebec Neuroblastoma Screening Project. *Pediatrics*, **86**, 765–73.

Woods, W.G., Tuchman, M., Robison, L.L., Bernstein, M., Léclerc, J.M., Brisson, L.C., Brossard, J., Hill, G., Shuster, J., Luepker, R., Byrne, T., Weitzman, S., Bunin, G. and Lemieux, B. (1996). A population-based study of the usefulness of screening for neuroblastoma. *Lancet*, **348**, 1682–7.

Index